OUTCOME MANAGEMENT AND PROGRAM EVALUATION MADE EASY: A TOOLKIT FOR OCCUPATIONAL THERAPY PRACTITIONERS

BY STEPHEN FORER, MA, MBA

The American Occupational Therapy Association, Inc.
Bethesda, MD

Disclaimers

"This publication is designed to provide accurate and authoritative information in regard to the subject matter covered. It is sold or distributed with the understanding that the publisher is not engaged in rendering legal, accounting, or other professional service. If legal advice or other expert assistance is required, the services of a competent professional person should be sought."

—From the Declaration of Principles jointly adopted by the American Bar Association and a Committee of Publishers and Associations

It is the objective of the American Occupational Therapy Association to be a forum for free expression and interchange of ideas. The opinions expressed by the contributors to this work are their own and not necessarily those of either the editors or the American Occupational Therapy Association.

ISBN 1-56900-038-7

Printed in the United States of America
Printed on recycled paper

TABLE OF CONTENTS

I. INTRODUCTION

II. MODELS OF OUTCOME EVALUATION

III. GENERAL ISSUES, TECHNIQUES, AND PROCEDURES FOR OUTCOME MANAGEMENT

ABOUT THE AUTHOR

Steve Forer, MA, MBA is a consultant in quality and outcome management, with extensive experience in business development, strategic planning, market research, systems design and analysis, and contract negotiations with managed care companies. He has operational experience with all levels of care in which rehabilitation services are provided. Formerly, he was the vice president of clinical outcomes management for NME, responsible for development and implementation of outcome measures, program evaluation, and continuous quality improvement in 34 free-standing rehabilitation hospitals, comprehensive outpatient centers, subacute facilities, and 35 acute care hospitals. Prior to joining NME, he was the vice president of patient care services for the Rehabilitation Hospital of the Pacific in Honolulu, Hawaii, and was responsible for overseeing the daily operations of all patient care departments in a 100-bed free-standing rehabilitation facility, comprehensive outpatient and satellite clinics. He presently serves as the co-chairperson of the National Advisory Committee for the Uniform Data System for Medical Rehabilitation (UDS). He was chairperson of the Data Sharing Committee and a past board member of the California Association of Rehabilitation Facilities. He was a member of the Health Care Financing Administration's Advisory Panel on Development of a Uniform Needs Assessment Instrument for Post Hospital Services.

Steve Forer has developed several outcome measures, including the Functional Assessment Measure (FAM). He has given numerous professional and scientific presentations in the areas of program evaluation, functional assessment, and management information systems, and has over 50 publications.

I. INTRODUCTION

The purpose of this resource guide is to provide a "practical toolkit" on outcome management and program evaluation for occupational therapy practitioners and to provide examples and applications related to all practice settings (i.e., acute care, acute rehabilitation, subacute rehabilitation, outpatient, home health, day treatment, mental health, and hand rehabilitation programs). This resource guide, which was developed under contract with The American Occupational Therapy Association (AOTA), explains three parallel but related concepts: outcome evaluation, quality management, and program evaluation as they relate to the practice of occupational therapy.

DIFFERENCES AND SIMILARITIES BETWEEN THREE PARALLEL AND RELATED CONCEPTS

OUTCOME EVALUATION

Outcome evaluation concentrates on the *results* of services, programs, treatments, or intervention strategies generally following termination of services or during a predetermined follow-up period. Outcome evaluation is a systematic procedure for monitoring the effectiveness and efficiency with which results are achieved following termination of services. Outcome evaluation generally focuses on the processes of care attributable to desired client outcomes, program performance, and the cost–benefits of outcomes achieved. An occupational therapy outcome is the functional consequence of the therapeutic intervention, such as independence in activities of daily living (ADL), return to work or former lifestyle, and general health perception. The World Health Organization (WHO, 1980[245]) has offered a conceptual framework for evaluating outcomes in terms of impact on *impairment, disability,* and *handicap.* According to AOTA's third edition of *Uniform Terminology for Occupational Therapy,* "achieving functional outcomes" means to develop, improve, or restore an individual to the highest possible level of independence. Function in terms of *performance areas* is the ultimate outcome objective for occupational therapy. Outcomes often can be used as a proxy to imply the quality of programs or services, but they are usually only a beginning point to help focus a quality improvement approach.

PROGRAM EVALUATION

Program evaluation is a much broader concept than outcome evaluation and may include needs assessment, process evaluation, program efficiency, program effectiveness, impact, and outcome evaluation, according to Weiss (1972).[103] The Commission on Accreditation of Rehabilitation

Facilities (CARF)[3, 187] has defined program evaluation as a "systematic procedure for determining the effectiveness and efficiency with which results are achieved by persons served during service delivery and following program completion, as well as the individual's satisfaction with them." Program evaluation management reports tell the facility whether its performance was acceptable according to goals and objectives that the facility/provider has established for itself. Since program evaluation includes outcome evaluation, the outcome measures used should relate to the overall program goals and objectives. There are two types of outcome measures described in Chapter 4: efficiency objectives and effectiveness objectives. In addition, program evaluation should include progress measures postdischarge, process measures that reflect the organizational goals in terms of strategic planning and program development, and measures of customer satisfaction. The main difference between program evaluation as defined by CARF and client-based outcome evaluation as defined by the Accreditation Council is that program evaluation tends to focus on the attainment of program results, whereas client-based outcome evaluation focuses on the attainment of individual client goals and outcome expectations. However, most program evaluators and program managers have considered the client's goals and outcome expectations, as well as comparative results from other providers in setting program goals, objectives, and expectancy levels.

QUALITY MANAGEMENT

Quality management is an even broader concept than program evaluation and generally encompasses all aspects of the organization and patient care. The Joint Commission on Accreditation of Health Care Organizations (JCAHO)[5] is shifting its focus from process to outcomes, while at the same time incorporating some of the concepts of total quality management, performance improvement, and business practices into its description of quality management. Quality management as defined by JCAHO is a planned, systematic, organizationwide approach to designing, measuring, assessing, and improving organizational performance in a multidisciplinary manner that monitors quality over the entire continuum of care and major organizational functions. There are 11 major (key) functions that can be divided into patient-focused functions and organization functions. Quality is assessed and managed in terms of efficacy of treatment, appropriateness of treatment, access or availability, timeliness, continuity, safety, efficiency, respect, and caring. Therefore, the scope of a quality management program, or performance improvement as outlined by JCAHO, tends to be a much more inclusive approach to determining the quality of programs or services provided. Since quality can be defined as meeting or exceeding the customer's expectations, it is important to survey the major customer groups (both internal and external customers) to identify their quality and outcome expectations so that these can be designed into a comprehensive quality management program. The provider or practitioner also needs to be prepared to deal with competing or conflicting customer expectations.

OVERVIEW OF THE BOOK

This guide provides an introduction to the preceding concepts, definitions of uniform terminology, emerging emphasis on outcomes and cost-effectiveness, utilization of results, applications for quality assurance/quality improvement, integration with other management information systems, accreditation, and reporting requirements (CARF, JCAHO, OBRA, Accreditation Council), identification of customers' outcome expectations, considerations in choosing/developing an outcome measure, examples of various program evaluation models, a description of commonly used outcome measures for each practice setting, methods of presenting and analyzing outcome results, data management and collection systems currently in use, key success factors, and future trends and directions. The "toolkit" is intended to provide practical examples and checklists, emphasize key points, and answer questions commonly asked about quality and outcome management. This resource guide is written for occupational therapy practitioners with a basic understanding of the subject areas.

II.
MODELS OF
OUTCOME EVALUATION

1. OVERVIEW OF OUTCOME EVALUATION

It is important for the reader to develop a clear understanding of the background and conceptual framework of outcome evaluation, and the growing importance of outcome evaluation in the health care industry. The next section of this resource guide provides readers with an overview of outcome evaluation in terms of

- a definition of outcome evaluation

- primary purposes of outcome evaluation

- the World Health Organization's (WHO) conceptional model of disablement with definitions of impairment, disability, and handicap

- a description of the American Occupational Therapy Association's (AOTA) *Uniform Terminology for Occupational Therapy* with definitions and examples of performance areas, performance components, and performance contexts

- a discussion of the emerging emphasis on outcomes and cost-effectiveness and the influence of managed care

- a discussion of the transition from quality assessment to performance improvement from the perspective of the Joint Commission on Accreditation of Healthcare Organizations (JCAHO) and the Accreditation Council on Services for People with Disabilities.

DEFINITION OF OUTCOME EVALUATION

Outcome evaluation concentrates on the results of services, programs, and treatment or intervention strategies generally following termination of services or during a predetermined follow-up period.[187] Outcome evaluation is a systematic procedure for monitoring the effectiveness and efficiency with which results are achieved by persons served as well as customer satisfaction following termination of services.[84] Outcome evaluation allows an evaluator, administrator, or program manager to systematically evaluate the outcome of rehabilitation efforts in terms of the operation, provision of services, appropriateness and effectiveness of services, efficiency of the system, and adequacy of serving the needs of the clients.[53] Some of the benefits a facility may gain through outcome evaluation are:

- identification of problem areas requiring more detailed investigation

- better alignment of internal program goals and objectives with client needs

- use of outcome data for research purposes

- cost-effectiveness information (the costs of a program are compared with the benefits or outcomes achieved by clients)

- informed decision making for future planning

- persuasive data for marketing purposes and contracting with managed care entities.

Despite these inherent benefits, the majority of occupational therapy practitioners resist doing outcome evaluation. This may be due in part to the lack of well-defined and tested outcome measures across the continuum of care. One purpose of this resource guide is to shed light on why the resistance exists, how it can be overcome, considerations in choosing/developing an outcome measure, and how to make outcome evaluation work
for you.

RATIONALE FOR USING OUTCOME EVALUATION

The main reasons for conducting outcome evaluation are to

- improve client benefits (effectiveness)

- improve efficiency (resource management)

- justify, maintain, or expand funding and general community support.

An occupational therapy outcome is the functional consequence for the patient of the therapeutic intervention by an occupational therapy practitioner. However, the temptation of many practitioners is to use refined clinical measures such as range of motion (ROM), muscle strength as measured by a dynamometer, endurance, or lifting and reaching capacity rather than measuring the actual functional outcome (i.e., independence in ADL, return to work or former lifestyle, quality of life, and general health perception). Although increased ROM, muscle strength, endurance, sensory and motor function, and cognitive and psychosocial function are all important, the key issue is what the patient is able to do (perform) as a result of these increased skills. If an increase of 10 percent in ROM does not appear to make any difference in a patient's ability to dress or feed himself or herself, then the intervention may not be perceived as cost-effective. Care should be taken in identifying the expected outcomes and measures for occupational therapy.

DEFINITIONS OF IMPAIRMENT, DISABILITY, AND HANDICAP

The term *function,* unfortunately, has many connotations. It may refer to an organ or system of the body, as in neuromuscular function, to task function as in dressing, or to the ability to function in a role that is socially expected, such as working or homemaking. The World Health Organization (WHO, 1980[245]) model of disablement and definitions of impairment, disability, and handicap provide a conceptual framework for evaluating outcomes and have become widely accepted by rehabilitation professionals and researchers.

> **Impairment** refers to "any loss or abnormality of psychological, physiological or anatomical structure or function." Examples of impairment would include the Impairment Groups from UDS$_{MR}$[39], nature and etiology of impairment, and Frankel (American Spinal Injury Association)[218] classification for spinal cord injury, range of motion (ROM), muscle tone and strength.

Disability refers to "any restriction or lack (resulting from an impairment) of ability to perform an activity in the manner or within the range considered normal for a human being." Disability refers to dysfunction of task performance. Examples include measures of severity of disability or burden of care such as the Functional Independence Measure (FIM)[39], activities of daily living (ADL), instrumental activities of daily living (IADL), and mobility, communication, cognitive, and psychosocial adjustment. Most of these measures are based on observed performance and not an assessment of capacity or capability.

Handicap refers to "a disadvantage for a given individual, resulting from an impairment or disability, that limits or prevents the fulfillment of a role that is normal for their [sic] age, gender and culture." The WHO definition of handicap includes six areas of role function: orientation, physical independence, mobility, occupation, social integration, and economic self sufficiency. Handicap is basically the social disadvantage of the impairment and resulting disability. Handicap measures might include work and productive activities, home management, educational and vocational activities, play and leisure, quality of life and perception of wellness.

A variety of different impairment, disability and handicap outcome measures may be selected for each occupational therapy practice setting. Most postacute, outpatient, work hardening, home health, and mental health program objectives tend to focus on the handicap issues, while the acute care, acute rehabilitation, and subacute program objectives tend to focus on impairment and disability issues.

USING UNIFORM TERMINOLOGY FOR OCCUPATIONAL THERAPY

AOTA has published its third edition of *Uniform Terminology for Occupational Therapy.*[244] According to this document, *occupational therapy* is the use of purposeful activity or intervention to promote health and achieve functional outcomes. "Achieving functional outcomes" means to develop, improve, or restore the highest possible level of independence of any individual who is limited by a physical injury or illness, a dysfunctional condition, a cognitive impairment, a psychological dysfunction, a mental illness, a developmental or learning disability, or an adverse environmental condition. Occupational therapy focuses on *performance areas, performance components,* and *performance contexts*.

Performance areas are broad categories of *human activity* that are typically part of daily life and include activities of daily living, work and productive activities, and play or leisure activities.

Performance components are fundamental *human abilities* that — to varying degrees and in different combinations — are required for successful engagement in performance areas. These components are sensorimotor, cognitive, psychosocial, and psychological.

Performance contexts are *situations or factors that influence* an individual's engagement in desired and/or performance areas. They may be temporal aspects (chronological, developmental, life cycle, and disability status) and environmental aspects (physical, social, and cultural).

Although function in *performance areas* is the ultimate objective of occupational therapy, function must be evaluated in light of the *performance components* and *performance contexts* that may have a direct impact on the outcomes in the performance areas. For example, a worker who is disabled from a work-related injury may have the potential for returning to work and productive activities. However, in order to accomplish this, the individual must first develop the strength, endurance, soft-tissue integrity, time management, and physical features of the performance contexts. It may be necessary to redesign the work tasks, adjust the work-load capacity, or provide vocational retraining or supported employment to enable the individual to return to work.

EMERGING EMPHASIS ON OUTCOMES AND COST-EFFECTIVENESS

Until fairly recently, the health care industry and occupational therapy practitioners have focused on the process of care, timeliness, and appropriateness of treatment. It only has been in the last 7 to 10 years that providers have begun to look more at outcomes. Third party payers, particularly managed care and workers' compensation carriers, have become increasingly concerned with long-term outcomes, total case costs, and future health care usage. Although several outcome measures have been developed for some practice settings, there is still a dearth of outcome measures across the continuum of care. There is no industry consensus over which tools to use or how to use them. In fact it may be a very unrealistic expectation to chose one outcome measure (gold standard) that is appropriate for all levels of care and practice settings. One thing is clear, however: providers must begin to evaluate the outcomes of their programs and services and to use this information to improve quality, outcomes, cost-effectiveness, and customer satisfaction. The goal of rehabilitation efforts has shifted from *maximizing functional recovery and independence* to *optimizing functional recovery,* transitioning patients as soon as possible, and—when it is safe to do so—to the least costly setting, thereby maximizing cost-effectiveness. Under a capitated health care system, providers will be forced to do just that.

TRANSITION FROM QUALITY ASSESSMENT TO PERFORMANCE IMPROVEMENT

In the past, quality assurance efforts have focused more on the processes of care and an audit-oriented retrospective approach to assessing quality of care. JCAHO is shifting its focus from process to outcomes, while at the same time trying to incorporate some total quality management, performance improvement, and business practices into a previously clinically dominant process system.[5] JCAHO's third initiative of the Agenda for Change focuses on incorporating outcomes and other performance measures in its future accreditation process. Individual providers are experiencing a paradigm shift as they continuously reevaluate their organizational structures, systems, and processes of care to gain further improvements in quality, outcome, and cost-effectiveness. The outcome and performance measures also must provide comparisons to external reference groups. The concept of performance improvement and patient-focused outcomes will be explained further in Chapter 5.

The Accreditation Council on Services for People with Disabilities, formerly the Accreditation Council on Services for People with Developmental Disabilities, began development of *Outcome Based Performance Measures* in 1991.[1] The council, which accredits 150 public and private agencies and programs in 23 states, has reduced their standards from 685 to 30 client-based outcome standards. These 30 standards now focus on a person's ability to choose personal goals and to actually achieve them. The choices may include living arrangements, work, leisure, community activities, friendships, relationships, privacy, and satisfaction with service providers. According to the Accreditation Council, outcome evaluation determines if individual client goals are achieved, whereas program evaluation determines whether program goals and objectives established by the clinical staff are obtained. ▪

2. USES OF OUTCOME EVALUATION

WHAT CAN OUTCOME EVALUATION DO FOR YOU

Outcome evaluation can have significant benefits for occupational therapy professionals, no matter what roles they fill—such as practitioner, faculty, administrator, or researcher in different practice settings. Outcome results presented in a concise, timely, understandable, and relevant manner can become a powerful management tool to assist in

- assessing quality
- modifying programs
- improving care for individual clients
- using outcome research for research
- conducting research on cost benefits
- determining functional recovery and level of care
- determining appropriateness of patient classification and payment systems
- planning for future program development
- marketing
- negotiating managed care contracts.

QUALITY ASSESSMENT PROGRAM MODIFICATION

The intention of outcome evaluation is to provide an overall picture of performance and outcome. In its simplest form, it does not provide specific answers to problem areas, but merely identifies that the problem exists.[53] By identifying problem areas, outcome evaluation can provide a more specific direction for performance improvement committees and may prompt individual chart audits or intensified studies to assist further in problem resolution.

Typical problems identified through various outcome studies include

- lack of anticipated improvement
- deterioration in functional abilities of clients
- preventable secondary medical complications
- excessive program costs or lengths of stay

- insufficient treatment

- substantial adjustment problems at home or in the community

- unexpected mortality

- rehospitalization

- poor motivation

- psychosocial maladjustment

- self-imposed social isolation

- discharge placement issues

- movement into more restrictive environments during follow-up

- regression to maladaptive behaviors

- inadequate use of community and outpatient services.[190]

PROGRAM MODIFICATION

As outcome information is processed and analyzed, suggestions frequently are made for the revision of existing programs, treatment techniques, or intervention strategies. One of the important benefits of outcome evaluation is that it allows a facility to monitor the impact of revised programs and techniques. It provides a baseline for comparing results before and after changes are made. Through this testing process, the most effective techniques can be selected and the treatment team can modify a program to better meet the needs of clients.

Outcome information can be very useful to the treatment staff. Most professionals dislike working in an environment in which standards used to evaluate their performance are unclear. Outcome evaluation can help by specifying the desired client outcomes. Also, through the use of outcome evaluation, management can provide staff with the resources needed to achieve desired results.

Results from outcome studies, both positive and negative, should be fed back to the entire staff. Such feedback can be encouraging to staff because it shows that client outcomes can be attributed directly to treatment. Studies have shown[38,106,110,116,119,123,136,143,156,186] that patients continue to improve after discharge from a comprehensive medical rehabilitation unit and that their functional level is typically higher than at discharge. Staff are concerned about what happens to their clients after treatment is completed. Although some patients may return for outpatient treatments, daycare treatment, or follow-up evaluations, at some facilities, the return rate is less than 40 percent of the inpatient caseload.[86] In addition to feedback on functional outcomes, staff often are interested in feedback on client satisfaction.

IMPROVING CARE FOR INDIVIDUAL CLIENTS

Outcome data can help OT professionals improve client care. When outcome data show that a specific client needs intervention, the professional can take prompt action to reduce the severity of the problem and resulting complications. To achieve this goal, criteria should be established for screening both inpatient and outpatient outcome data to trigger immediate review of the potential problem by the appropriate person. Screening criteria should be developed to identify patients who are having substantial adjustment problems at home, have developed secondary medical complications, or have deteriorated in functional status. This information can then be relayed to the appropriate team members for corrective action or follow-up services. In one study[119], approximately 17 percent of the former rehabilitation inpatients were identified with such problems and 10 percent were readmitted for inpatient rehabilitation. Other follow-up action may include increased in-home health services, outpatient therapy, patient/family education, or referral to the appropriate medical profession.

USING OUTCOME DATA FOR RESEARCH

Outcome evaluation can be useful for research and comparative studies. Special studies often are needed to further refine outcome information for management purposes. Outcome data can be regrouped and compared according to various factors. Some common types of comparative analyses of functional outcomes include

- clients receiving different durations or intensity of treatment

- clients experiencing different treatment techniques or in different practice settings

- clients being discharged home as opposed to long-term-care facilities

- treatment occurring during different quarters of the year (3-month intervals)

- some clients receiving comprehensive rehabilitation services and others receiving less-intensive services.

Some investigators have used functional outcome data in attempts to identify the best predictors of successful outcome for disabled persons following rehabilitation. Several studies have shown that the age at onset and duration of initial hospitalization tend to be the best predictors.[24,38,110,131,150,153] Another study[119] suggests that bladder management and cognition are the best predictors of successful home placement. Several studies[6,10,14,15,122,153] have shown that duration of coma and time from onset to rehabilitation admission are the best predictors of functional recovery and outcome for individuals with traumatic brain injury. Others[117,126,127,144,145,150,154] have related the findings of computerized axial tomography (CAT) to the prediction of functional recovery following a stroke or head injury. One recent study[121] found that neurobehavioral responsiveness to be predictive of short-term outcomes in minimally responsive head trauma patients. Another study[142] related carotid artery occlusion to stroke outcomes. Still other studies[129,147] have related levels of distress, agitation, and restlessness to head injury outcomes.

Similar attempts have been made to identify the best predictors of functional recovery in other rehabilitation settings. In one study[235], the factor consistently related to patient outcomes in nursing homes was RN hours. Another study[241] examined predictors of mortality in nursing homes versus community residents. The presence of a spouse at home, number of previous admissions, mental disorder, and musculoskeletal disorder also have been found to be important predictors of successful home placement for nursing home residents.[238] In drug and alcohol treatment programs studies have found social class, age, education, employment history, and marital status to be related to treatment outcomes. All of the aforementioned are examples of how outcome data can be used for research or comparison purposes.

CONDUCTING RESEARCH ON COST–BENEFITS

One very important area of research is the cost-effectiveness and cost–benefits of rehabilitation. There appears to be favorable evidence of the cost–benefits of stroke and head injury rehabilitation, and stronger evidence of the cost-effectiveness in spinal cord injury rehabilitation.[130] The benefits of early rehabilitation have been demonstrated for head injury[6,153] and stroke patients.[131] However, there has been little published on this subject since the early 1980s. Most of the studies lack adequate control groups. Outcomes between practice settings and types of rehabilitation programs need to be compared. One controversial study[132] found that increased intensity of therapy services (PT and OT) as a result of the Medicare Three Hour Rule, did not necessarily lead to better outcomes but added to the costs of rehabilitation. Another study found that there was little correlation between FIM[SM] gains and therapy hours.[185] Further research is desperately needed in this area.

FUNCTIONAL RECOVERY AND LEVEL OF CARE DETERMINATIONS

Functional outcomes and progress measures should be used not only in the initial level of care determinations, but also in deciding when to move a patient to the next level of care. Research on functional outcomes can provide some guidance on the key decision points. The goal of rehabilitation, regardless of practice setting, has shifted away from the traditional goal of maximizing functional outcome, to a more pragmatic goal of optimizing functional recovery. Under a capitated reimbursement system, providers will be forced to move patients efficiently through the continuum of care. There is a point of diminishing returns when a patient's progress and recovery are not as rapid as in previous days or weeks. It is at this point that the treatment team needs to consider moving the patient to a lower, less costly setting to maximize cost-effectiveness.

DETERMINING APPROPRIATE PATIENT CLASSIFICATION AND PAYMENT SYSTEMS

FUNCTION-RELATED GROUPS

The current Medicare prospective payment system (DRGs) has not been found to be an appropriate payment system for rehabilitation.[171,175,185] However, functional status upon admission and discharge from rehabilitation shows promise in being able to predict resource consumption (rehabilitation length of stay [LOS] and costs). A patient classification system (FIM[SM]–FRGs) has been developed by Stineman et al.[181,182] to classify medical rehabilitation patients into homogeneous LOS, and as a possible basis for a prospective payment system for inpatient acute rehabilitation. Fifty-three FRGs were developed based on the Rehabilitation Impairment Categories (RIC), functional status on admission (FIM[SM] motor and cognitive subscores), and patient's age, which explained over 40 percent of the variance in LOS in the combined validation and modeling samples. This is more than twice the amount of variance initially explained by the DRGs. Stineman and colleagues[183] also have examined different variations of the FRGs using the individual FIM^{SM} items, the clinical subscales (i.e. self care, sphincter control, mobility transfers, mobility locomotion, communication, and social-cognition) and the total FIM^{SM} scores. Further research is needed to refine the FRGs, identify LOS outliers, include comorbidities/complications, provide a methodology for calculating relative weights, case-mix adjustments, facility payment adjustors (i.e., cost outliers, transfers back to acute care, program interruptions), and other economic factors.

It is important to recognize that FRGs are a patient classification system, not a payment or reimbursement model. A payment model could be developed with relative weights based on:

- a refined version of the FRGs, with adjustors similar to those used in DRGs

- FRGs plus facility and economic adjustors

- quality incentive pool based on an overall performance index (FIM^{SM} change, LOS, percent discharged to community, and case-mix/severity adjustor)

- some other alternative system.

The American Rehabilitation Association (ARA) has developed a proposal for a Medicare Prospective Payment System for Rehabilitation Hospitals and Units[178], using an FRG approach to payment modeling.[42] The Health Care Financing Administration (HCFA) has awarded a grant to the RAND Corporation to evaluate case classification systems and design a prospective payment system for inpatient rehabilitation. The study is expected to be completed by September 1996. In the meantime, ARA is pursuing rebasing the TEFRA limits for the exempt rehabilitation hospitals and units, and 305 of the current UDS subscribers have agreed to release their facility data to HCFA for inclusion in the study.

AMBULATORY PATIENT CLASSIFICATION SYSTEM

A similar patient classification and payment system is being developed for ambulatory care. The 3M Health Information Systems has been contracted by HCFA to develop an Ambulatory Patient Classification System (APGs) designed to explain the amount and type of resources used in ambulatory care.[170] APGs were developed to encompass the full range of ambulatory settings, including surgery units, hospital emergency rooms, outpatient clinics, and day hospitals. A total of 289 APGs have been identified based on the Major Diagnostic Categories (MDCs) from the DRG classification system, CPT codes, Relative Value Units (RVUs), and Signs, Symptoms and Findings (SSFs). The APGs performed 58 percent better than the DRGs in predicting ambulatory resource consumption. A series of V-Codes, H-Codes, and SSFs have been developed. The H-Codes, which include a section on Functional Health Status, are intended for use in reporting the functional status of rehabilitation patients, mental patients, and patients with chronic illnesses in all ambulatory settings. The functional status items and rating scales are based on a modification of the Patient Evaluation Conference System (PECs)[26], which has not been widely tested for ambulatory settings. Further research is being conducted by 3M and the New York State Department of Health to refine and validate the APG model. It is likely that similar systems to the FRGs and APGs will eventually be developed for psychiatric care, children's hospitals, long-term hospitals, home health, and longterm care.

PLANNING FOR FUTURE PROGRAM DEVELOPMENT

Outcome data can be used for planning future program development as well as projecting various growth rates or changes in client programs. Outcome evaluation provides a basis for monitoring changes in variables such as:

- client characteristics or needs
- diagnostic composition of caseload
- number of clients treated
- number of treatments rendered per patient
- average length of treatment
- average cost per case
- program interruptions
- age of clientele
- sex and race distribution
- referral patterns
- time from onset of disability to rehabilitation treatment
- utilization of outpatient or other community services.

When these types of outcome and descriptive data are effectively integrated with various management information systems (such as productivity statistics, revenue statistics, staffing, census, and daily treatment records), projecting a growth rate based on retrospective and concurrent data is possible. Facility-based planners and health care consultants have used acute care discharge statistics, prevalence and incidence models to predict demand for and utilization of services in a variety of settings including acute rehabilitation, subacute care, outpatient therapy, and home health programs. Table 1 provides an example of how an incidence-based model might be used to predict occupational therapy visits for stroke patients in different practice settings for a given service area. However, local market conditions, possible variations in incidence rates and population growth rates, age distribution, and competition from other providers must be taken into consideration. The five-year forecast adjusts for age cohorts, changing utilization patterns, declining LOS, and the influence of managed care.

MARKETING OT PROGRAMS AND SERVICES

One of the major purposes of outcome evaluation is to justify, maintain, or expand funding and general community support. Outcome data can be helpful in marketing occupational therapy programs and services to current and potential referral sources and clientele, as well as in promoting better community awareness and acceptance. The Commission on Accreditation of Rehabilitation Facilities (CARF)[3], the Accreditation Council[1], and even to some extent the Joint Commission on Accreditation of Healthcare Organizations[5] have advocated utilization of outcome

TABLE 1.
PROJECTIONS OF FUTURE UTILIZATION
ESTIMATES OF NEED, DEMAND, AND SUPPLY FOR
STROKE REHABILITATION

Stroke Programs (OT)	1994 Based Year	1999 5-Year Forecast
Service Area Population (primary & secondary)	540,000	588,600
Incidence Rate (per 1,000 population)	1.6490	1.9778
Estimated number of cases	890	1,164
Survival Rate (92%)	819	1,071
Survivors Appropriate for:		
Acute Rehab (40%)	327	428
Subacute (61%)	500	652
Outpatient (63%)	516	675
Home Health (45%)	369	482
Estimated Duration of Treatment:		
Acute Care ALOS	11	9
Acute Rehab ALOS	24	22
Subacute ALOS	23	22
Outpatient OT Visits/Patient	18	18
Home Health OT Visits/Patient	18	18
Inpatient Program Days:		
Acute Care	9,009	9,639
Acute Rehab	7,848	9,416
Subacute	11,500	14,344
Estimated Demand for OT: (30 minute increments)		
Acute Care OT Visits	2,455	3,213
Acute Rehab OT Visits	19,060	24,947
Subacute OT Visits	20,700	26,993
Outpatient OT Visits	9,288	12,150
Home Health OT Visits	6,642	8,676
Provider Utilization: (30 minute increments)		
Acute Care OT Visits	1,050	1,415
Acute Rehab OT Visits	8,005	9,980
Subacute OT Visits	4,140	4,858
Outpatient OT Visits	2,322	2,795
Home Health OT Visits	1,993	2,430
Market Share:		
Acute Care OT	43%	44%
Acute Rehab OT	41%	40%
Subacute OT	20%	18%
Outpatient OT	25%	23%
Home Health OT	30%	28%

and quality results in marketing programs and services to external groups and third party payers. The outcome claims, however, must be valid, reliable, honest, and consistent with data contained in the provider's internal management information and program evaluation systems.

COMPARING PROGRAMS

To market an occupational therapy program effectively and to enhance the image of the program in the community, it is helpful to know the costs, lengths of treatment, and functional outcome of various conditions treated in the program and how these figures compare to similar programs or to different types of settings that may also treat the same type of clientele. However, there are often differences in the type and intensity of services provided, philosophy and goals of the program, staffing patterns, and acuity or severity of disabilities and conditions treated that can affect both costs and outcome. Having an overall sense of the characteristic differences between programs and care settings is essential. Elaborate and appropriate comparative data are needed so that sound marketing decisions can be made.[189,190] Outcome results must be compared with similar providers and external reference groups. The health care reform movement and development of provider report cards eventually will force providers to compare their results and share them with the general public.

Uniform Data System for Medical Rehabilitation (UDS$_{MR}$) has established a Policy for the Release of Facility Data[100] to ensure that comparisons are accurate, valid, appropriate, and not misleading (see below).

POLICY FOR RELEASING FACILITY DATA

- Facility must be a current UDS$_{MR}$ subscriber.

- Facility must be fully credentialed (passed Phases 1 and 2 of UDS Credentialing).

- Facility must submit a full calendar year's data for all patients in reported impairment groups.

- Facility must evaluate case mix differences and only compare within impairment groups.

- Statistical parameters such as facility standard deviations are to be reported.

- The UDS$_{MR}$ Facility Report and reporting period must be referenced.

- A facility may compare its results with UDS$_{MR}$ national figures published in the *American Journal of Physical Medicine and Rehabilitation* but must cite the appropriate article.

- Care should be taken when making greater than or less than comparisons to include standard deviations and statistical significance of the differences.

Other comparable data management services such as Formations in Health Care[51], have established similar criteria to ensure accurate and honest comparisons with other providers. Training and credentialing processes have been established to ensure adequate interrater reliability and accuracy of function outcome scores reported. Despite such efforts, some providers have chosen to collect, analyze, and report their own functional outcome results without participating in a data management service and subjecting their data to this scrutiny. Such outcome claims, unless substantiated, may be false and misleading.

PRESENTING OUTCOME DATA

Outcome information should be presented in a simple format that is easily understood. The use of graphs and tables can be helpful to display functional outcome, duration of treatment, and costs of rehabilitation by disability, as well as percentages of different discharge dispositions. Often a narrative summary also is beneficial. Facilities may wish to publish quarterly or annual outcome information for marketing purposes. Figures 1–8, show how some of this information can be presented graphically for marketing purposes. A facility's outcome results are compared with UDS_MR national averages, and a system of managed rehabilitation units in acute care hospitals.

NEGOTIATING CONTRACTS WITH MANAGED CARE PROVIDERS

Many providers have begun to use their outcome and quality results in contract negotiations with managed care entities. These results are used to provide evidence of the clinical expertise of treating staff, track record with past patient outcomes, and some comparison to other providers. Large group health plans and managed care plans have become increasingly interested in total case costs, long-term outcomes, future health care utilization, and how rehabilitation has saved them money in the long run. This has significant implications for most providers, who are focusing their outcome evaluation and management systems entirely around what happens to patients while they are under treatment. It is rare for providers to collect any outcome information beyond 6–9 months after termination of treatment. Thus they are not in a very good position to answer the questions many managed care companies are raising, namely long-term outcomes, maintenance of functional gains, subsequent health care use, and costs related to a patient's disability. This implies that outcome information should be collected as long as 1–2 years after termination of services to meet payers' needs. Cost-effective methods of collecting long-term outcomes are explored in Chapter 7 of this resource guide. ■

FIGURE 1.

Rehab Caseload

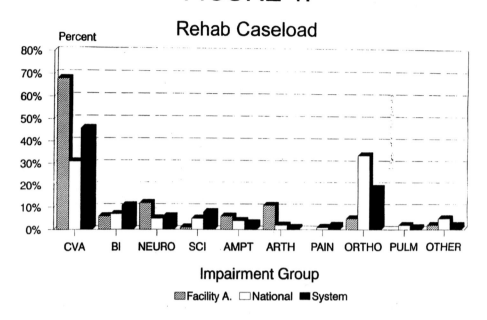

UDS Report of First Admits for 1993, American Journal of Physical Med. 74 (1), Feb. 1995.

FIGURE 2.

Rehab ALOS

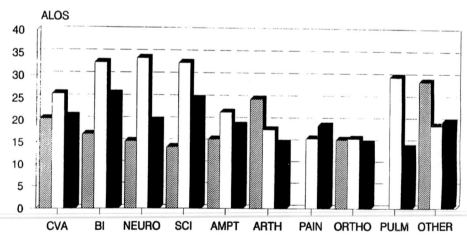

UDS Report of First Admits for 1993, American Journal of Physical Med, 74 (1) Feb. 1995

FIGURE 3.

% D/C to Community

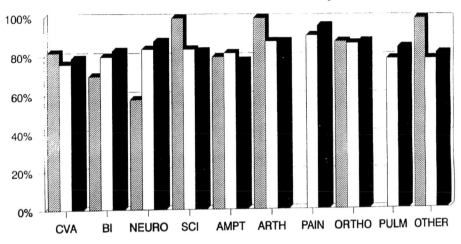

Impairment Group

Facility A.   National   System

UDS Report of First Admits for 1993, American Journal of Physical Med., 74 (1), Feb. 1995

FIGURE 4.

Admission FIM

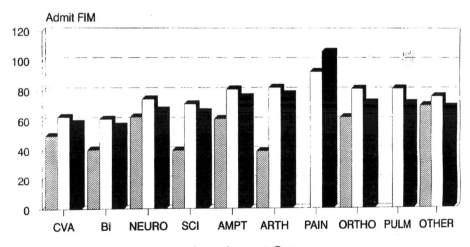

Impairment Group

Facility A.   National   System

UDS Report of First Admits for 1993, American Journal of Physical Med., 74 (1), Feb. 1995.

FIGURE 5.

Discharge FIM

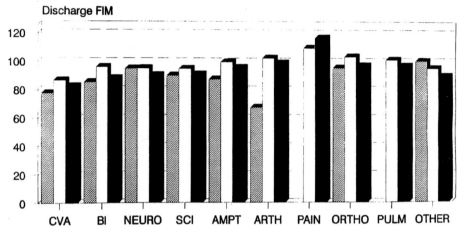

UDS Report of First Admits for 1993, American Journal of Physical Med., 74 (1), Feb. 1995.

FIGURE 6.

FIM Change

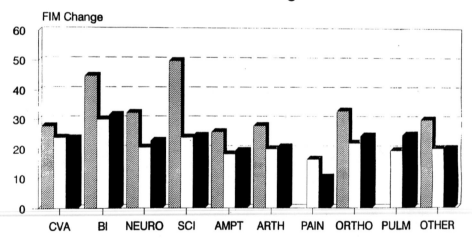

UDS Report of First Admits for 1993, American Journal of Physical Med., 74 (1), Feb. 1995.

FIGURE 7.

LOS Efficiency (FIM gain/LOS)

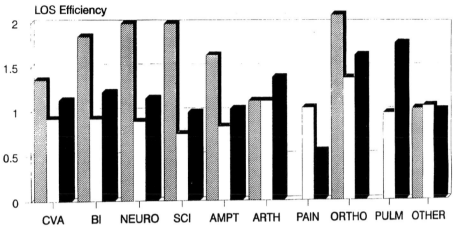

UDS Report of First Admits for 1993, American Journal of Physical Med., 74 (1), Feb. 1995

FIGURE 8.

FOLLOW-UP FIM (6 months)

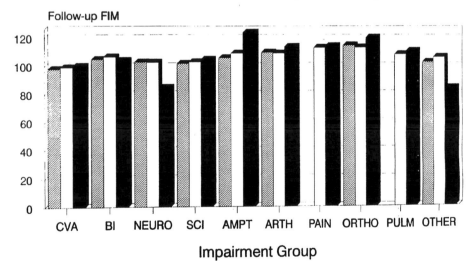

UDS Report #1 for First Admiits for 1993

3. OVERVIEW OF PROGRAM EVALUATION

WHAT IS PROGRAM EVALUATION?

In the current cost-conscious climate, programs must show that they are delivering what they promise. Program evaluation is a means for administrators and managers to demonstrate that their program is achieving its goals. Program evaluation is a much broader concept than outcome evaluation and may include needs assessment, process evaluation, program efficiency, and impact and outcome evaluation, according to Weiss (1972).[103]

This chapter provides a definition of program evaluation according to the Commission on Accreditation of Rehabilitation Facilities (CARF) and CARF's requirements for program evaluation. CARF is a voluntary accreditation agency for organizations serving persons with disabilities and has accredited over 1,800 such organizations including comprehensive inpatient rehabilitation, spinal cord injury, brain injury, chronic pain, early intervention and preschool development, substance abuse and chemical dependency, mental health, and psychosocial rehabilitation programs.

DEFINITION OF PROGRAM EVALUATION

Although the concept of program evaluation started in the mental health field over 30 years ago, CARF's definition is the most useful because it focuses on rehabilitation programs. In CARF's 1995 *Standards Manual*[3,187], "*program evaluation* is a systematic procedure for determining the effectiveness and efficiency with which results are achieved by persons served both during service delivery and following program completion as well as the individual's satisfaction with them." Program evaluation management reports tell the facility/provider whether its performance is acceptable according to the goals, objectives, and expectancy levels that the facility/provider has established for itself.

HOW IS PROGRAM EVALUATION DIFFERENT FROM CLIENT-BASED OUTCOME EVALUATION?

The main difference between program evaluation and client-based outcome evaluation is that program evaluation tends to focus on the attainment of program results, whereas client-based outcome evaluation focuses on the attainment of client goals and outcome expectations. However, most evaluators and program directors have considered the client's goals and outcome expectations, as well as comparative results from other providers, in setting the program's goals, objectives, and expectancy levels.

RATIONALE FOR USING PROGRAM EVALUATION

Program evaluation as defined by CARF is a systematic procedure for determining the effectiveness of results achieved by persons served during service delivery or after program completion and measuring the individual's satisfaction with those results. A program evaluation system should measure outcomes, progress, and process of care delivery and how well the persons served are functioning after termination of services. This implies that some follow-up measures will be included in the program evaluation system. The reports produced from a program evaluation system tell the facility or provider whether its performance was acceptable according to goals and objectives that the facility or provider has established for itself.

The program evaluation results should be presented in a clear, understandable, and concise manner to program managers, administrators, governing bodies, medical staff, third party payers, referring professionals and agencies, potential consumers, and the community. Any individual or agency who may be in a position to make decisions or influence program performance should have access to the program evaluation results.

RATIONALE FOR USING CARF STANDARDS

The CARF Standards provide an excellent and comprehensive framework for conducting, communicating, and using program evaluation for planning and modifying programs and services and for marketing and program promotion. CARF encourages organizations to use their program evaluation results in their marketing brochures and material. However, the information contained in these brochures must be accurate and consistent with current results of the program evaluation system. Most of the CARF-accredited organizations have been able to effectively use their program evaluation results to demonstrate program improvements to external customers and to guide the development of new programs and services. CARF has produced a number of publications to assist facilities and providers in the development and utilization of the program evaluation systems.

CARF REQUIREMENTS FOR PROGRAM EVALUATION

CARF guidelines cover the essential elements, program components, management reports, and minimum requirements for each program type.

ESSENTIAL ELEMENTS OF PROGRAM EVALUATION

According to CARF's 1995 *Standards Manual* (p. 57 3a), there are four elements that must be included in a program evaluation system, as follows:

1. a purpose/mission statement for the organization

2. a program structure delineating all major programs and product lines

3. a system review mechanism

4. management reports.

PROGRAM COMPONENTS

These essential program components must relate to the overall purpose and mission of the organization, the program structure (delineating major programs or product lines), and the system review mechanisms. According to the CARF manual (p. 57 3a2), for each identified program, there must be:

- a goal statement
- admission criteria
- a listing of services offered
- measurable objectives
- measurement criteria (outcome measures)
  efficiency measures
  effectiveness measures
  measures of customer satisfaction
- specification of to whom measure is applied
- specification of time each measure is applied
- priority ranking or weights for each objective
- specification of characteristics of persons served (client descriptors)
- follow-up information.

MANAGEMENT REPORTS

The final essential part of the process is the management report. These reports tell the facility and providers whether their performance met the goals and objectives that the facility has established. The results should be clear, concise, timely, understandable, and relevant to those receiving the information. Outcome information should be presented to program managers, administrators, governing bodies, third party payers, referring professionals and agencies, potential consumers, and the community. Those persons and organizations who are in a position to make decisions and facilitate change or improve performance and outcome should have access to outcome information.

According to the CARF manual (p. 58 3a4), the management reports should include:

- measures of effectiveness
- measures of efficiency
- measures of customer satisfaction
- characteristics of persons served
- interpretation of results.

The results of the program evaluation should be made available to decision makers as soon as possible (not more than 120 days after the end of the reporting period), and should be used to improve quality and program performance. The results should be reviewed by the entire treatment team to identify problem areas, trends, possible extraneous variables and explanations, recommendations, and action plans. Although the team members may not be the final decision makers, they often can add useful insight in interpreting the findings. Once the reports have been reviewed by the treatment team, they can be passed on to other review committees with comments and recommendations (CARF 1995 manual, p. 59 3c).

PROGRAM EVALUATION REQUIREMENTS FOR DIFFERENT TYPES OF PROGRAMS

CARF provides specific requirements for program evaluation for various types of programs, including medical rehabilitation, comprehensive inpatient, outpatient medical rehabilitation, occupational rehabilitation, comprehensive pain management, brain injury, community employment, and early intervention and preschool developmental programs, as shown below.

CARF REQUIREMENTS FOR SPECIFIC PROGRAMS

Medical Rehabilitation Programs (CARF 1995 *Standards Manual,* p. 66 A.7)

- functional outcomes

- medical outcomes

- disposition at discharge

- status of postdischarge functional abilities

- patient/family satisfaction.

The functional outcomes should be related to effectiveness measures. The medical outcomes should be related to the medical status of the patient such as control of diabetes, cardiac, or pulmonary function. Data on postdischarge status should be gathered for all persons served. Follow-up outcome information should be collected at different time intervals for various impairment groups (e.g., brain injury at 2 weeks, 1, 2, 3, and 6 months postdischarge; spinal cord injury at 3 weeks, 6 weeks, 3 and 6 months; orthopedic 1-2 weeks, 3 and 6 months). Program evaluation data should be collected 80-180 days postdischarge.

COMPREHENSIVE INPATIENT

In addition to the program evaluation standards under medical rehabilitation programs, the program evaluation system for Comprehensive Inpatient, Categories 1-3, should also include the following:

- the percentage of unplanned transfer to acute medical facilities

- the percentage of patients who achieved discharge criteria (goals)

- the percentage of patients discharged to long-term care

- the percentage of patients who expire.

Most hospital-based subacute rehabilitation programs will fall into Category 2 of Comprehensive Inpatient Rehabilitation, in which the patients have a variable risk of potential medical instability, complex medical conditions, and are receiving an average of 1 to 3 hours of therapy at least 5 days per week. Therefore, it is important to carefully monitor medical conditions that may cause a program interruption and/or transfer back to an acute care facility. The nursing acuity system should relate to the rehabilitation and medical needs of the patients and the amount of nursing care required.

OUTPATIENT MEDICAL REHABILITATION.

The following requirements are in addition to those for medical rehabilitation:

- degree of accomplishment of functional goals

- status of postdischarge functional abilities

- patient/family satisfaction.

OCCUPATIONAL REHABILITATION PROGRAMS

- progress toward functional, work-related goals

- frequency, duration, and costs of services

- work capability at discharge

- status of postdischarge functional, work-related abilities.

WORK-SPECIFIC OCCUPATIONAL REHABILITATION PROGRAMS

The following requirements are in addition to those for occupational rehabilitation programs:

- percentage of persons returning to work

- percentage of persons receiving vocational services

- percentage of persons receiving other services

- percentage of persons returning to their original jobs.

COMPREHENSIVE PAIN MANAGEMENT

In addition to those measures listed under medical rehabilitation, the program evaluation system for chronic comprehensive pain management must include at least two of the following:

- return to work when appropriate

- appropriate use of medication

- decreased intensity of subjective pain

- increased ability to manage pain

- increased functional activities

Comprehensive pain management may include inpatient and outpatient programs, or outpatient programs only, for chronic and cancer-related pain conditions. In addition, the cancer-related comprehensive pain management program evaluation system must include a measure of quality of life.

BRAIN-INJURY PROGRAMS

In addition to the requirements under medical rehabilitation, a program evaluation system for brain injury postacute and community integrated programs must include:

- degree of personal and living independence

- level of work productivity

- psychological and social adjustment.

COMMUNITY EMPLOYMENT SERVICES

The program evaluation system for community employment services should include:

- average number of consecutive weeks worked

- average number of hours worked per week

- earnings and benefits

- job retention

- job advancement

- job changes

- length of time from referral to placement

- type and amount of staff intervention

- integration

- number of successful placements

- satisfaction of employer with services provided.

EARLY INTERVENTION AND PRESCHOOL DEVELOPMENTAL PROGRAMS

- number of children who have no need for further specialized services

- level of integration into appropriate community settings

- movement into less restrictive environments

- family's satisfaction with the program

- developmental gains as measured by standardized tools

- attainment of individual program goals objectives

- level of family participation

4. SPECIFIC PROCEDURES FOR PROGRAM EVALUATION

A number of specific steps and techniques are necessary in order to implement a program evaluation. This section provides examples of the various parts of the process, including selecting efficiency and effectiveness objectives, determining client descriptors, establishing relative weights, calculating standard or program index scores, and developing program evaluation matrices for comprehensive inpatient rehabilitation, subacute, and outpatient medical rehabilitation programs.

SETTING UP A PROGRAM EVALUATION SYSTEM

In the development of a program evaluation system, a sample of the efficiency and effectiveness objectives, client descriptors, and supplemental measures are selected that meets the clinical and management staff's need for information and that matches the overall goals of the program. Outcome objectives are also selected on the basis of the customer's expectations, namely, the patient, family members, referring physician, case manager, managed care company, worker's compensation carrier, or other third party payer.

The first step is to choose the relevant efficiency and effectiveness objectives, based on the program goals and client descriptors, and then weight these objectives in terms of their relative importance. Next, expectancy levels must be determined for each objective. Then, an index score conversion table must be developed to convert raw scores to index scores for each objective so that a single performance index score ultimately can be determined for the program. Examples of program evaluation systems are shown in Appendices A, B, and C.

EFFICIENCY AND EFFECTIVENESS OBJECTIVES

An efficiency objective measures how resources (inputs) are used to achieve the program goals. Efficiency objectives commonly used in program evaluation systems for various rehabilitation programs are shown below.

An effectiveness objective measures the extent to which the program has achieved various outcomes (outputs). A large variety of effectiveness objectives have been used in different program evaluation systems. Some examples are shown on the following page.

EXAMPLES OF EFFICIENCY OBJECTIVES

average cost/case (i.e., cost containment)

average duration of treatment (ALOS, number of visits or weeks)

average number of daily treatment hours

maximize service efficiency (i.e., LOS efficiency, functional gain/number of treatments)

timeliness of treatment

appropriate level of care utilization

percent of clients completing program

EXAMPLES OF EFFECTIVENESS OBJECTIVES

increase/maximize self-care skills

increase/maximize mobility skills

increase/maximize communication skills

increase/maximize psychosocial adjustment

increase cognitive function

facilitate community reintegration

secure recommended services

percent discharged home

avoid institutionalization

enhance social adjustment

increase participation in social activities

enhance family relationships

minimize accidents at home

minimize preventable medical complications

maximize bowel/bladder management (continence)

enhance caregiver training/family education

maximize satisfaction with services rendered (required by CARF)

decrease agitation

improve judgment and reasoning abilities

maximize vocational independence

maintain functional gains acquired (following completion of program)

increase strength, endurance, and coordination

increase functional work capacity

prevent reinjury

return to gainful employment

minimize health care use related to injury

reduce reliance on pain medications

decrease subjective pain

increase ability to manage pain

attainment of functional and/or program goals

Most outcome evaluation systems consist of no more than 10 primary effectiveness and efficiency objectives.[190] Each of these objectives must be weighted in terms of its relative importance with respect to the other objectives. Some of the objectives may be applied during the program and others after termination of services. It may be helpful to separate the program outcome results from the follow-up outcome results, and to produce two separate management reports, one for each time frame. The advantages of this approach is that the program evaluation (PE) management report can be produced more quickly, and results are more easily traceable to treatment interventions.[84,120] Also, patients who expire or are unable to be contacted during follow-up may be included in the first PE management report reflecting performance and outcome while they were in the program, but are excluded from the follow-up report.

CLIENT DESCRIPTORS

It is important to describe the demographics of any patient study sample. Client descriptors are important to include in a program evaluation system because they can often help to explain variance from expected performance on many of the efficiency or effectiveness measures. In addition, there may be changes in client characteristics or needs, as indicated by the client descriptors, which may require program modifications or expanded services. In program evaluation, demographics are usually referred to as *client descriptors,* which are statements that define the population in terms of the severity of problems or barriers to individual success. Examples of frequently reported client descriptors are shown below.

EXAMPLES OF CLIENT DESCRIPTORS

average age and breakdown by age groups
sex distribution
race distribution
payment source
referral source
average number of hospital days before rehabilitation
average time from onset to rehabilitation admission
circumstances of onset
percent with prior medical complications (comorbidities)
percent who had surgery
percent transferred back to acute care
percent who expire
number of subsequent hospitalizations
geographic distribution
percent employed/student prior to onset

ESTABLISHING EXPECTANCY LEVELS

Expectancy levels or thresholds are established for each selected measure and program objective based on past provider performance and comparison to other providers. CARF[187] has suggested establishing three expectancy levels for each program object:

- *Minimum* (threshold below which performance should never drop),

- *Goal* (target performance level based on past experience or external reference group), and

- *Optimal* (the best expected performance in the context of the population served and scope of the program — rarely set at 100 percent).

These expected levels are reviewed continuously and updated to reflect increased performance capabilities. The intervals between the minimum (e.g., 70 percent), goal (e.g., 80 percent) and optimal expectancies (e.g., 95 percent) do not necessarily need to be the same. Specific expectancy levels may be established for each major impairment group (e.g., stroke, neurological, musculoskeletal, and other) for some objectives. In contrast to the CARF model, JCAHO suggests establishing two expectancy levels: threshold (minimum acceptable performance) and target level (goal for each indicator based on best practices and external reference groups).

WEIGHTING PROGRAM OBJECTIVES

Each program objective is then weighted in terms of its relative importance compared with the other objectives. For example, if you had 10 program objectives that were equally weighted, each would be worth 10 percent. However, this is rarely the case, and some program objectives are clearly more important then others. One useful method is to use the nominal group process with the treatment team and external customers to help prioritize the program objectives. Have each member rate the importance of each objective on a 1 to 10 point scale, (where 10 = extremely important and 1 = not important). Take an average of the importance ratings on each program objective from the group members, and prioritize the objectives from highest ratings to the lowest ratings. Then take 100 percent and split it up among the program objectives to reflect this priority or sequence. As you can see in the following example, some of the objectives may be closely rated in terms of relative importance and therefore receive the same relative weight.

OBJECTIVE #	IMPORTANCE RANKING	RELATIVE WEIGHT
1	9.25	14%
2	9.00	13%
3	8.75	12%
4	8.50	11%
5	8.25	10%
6	8.00	9%
7	7.95	9%
8	7.50	8%
9	7.45	8%
10	7.00	6%
Total	**8.16**	**100%**

INDEX SCORE CONVERSION TABLES

In order to establish a single standard score or performance index score for a program, you need to create an index score conversion table (matrix) to convert actual results in raw scores to index scores for each program objective. This is important so one can get an overall assessment of program performance across all program objectives and over time. The *Optimal* expectancy level can be assigned an index score of 150 points, *Goal* 100 points, and *Minimal* expectancy level 50 points. Using the expectancy levels for each objective, you can create a matrix of index score equivalents for each possible raw score between the optimal, goal, and minimum expectancy level as shown in Table 2. The mathematical formula is as follows: (*Optimal* expectancy—*Goal* expectance level)/ 50 points (the difference between the index score equivalent for Optimal 150 and the index score for Goal 50) = unit change in raw score for each increment of 1 index score equivalent. The product would be multiplied by 5 and subtracted from the *Optimal* expectancy for each decrease of 5 index points. For example, if the optimal expectancy level of objective #2 was 90 percent, and the goal expectancy was 80 percent, there would be a 5 point drop in index score for each 1 percent decrease in actual raw score (90 percent-80 percent)/50 X's 5 = 1%. So an actual raw score of 85 percent would equal an index score of 125, as shown in Table 2. The same procedure would be used to establish index score equivalents for incremental changes in raw scores between the *Goal* and *Minimum* expectancy levels. With the assistance of computer spreadsheets, this process can be made much simpler. Another approach used by providers is to simply take the actual raw score as a percentage of the target or Goal expectancy level. In the previous example if the actual result was 85 percent, then the index score would be 1.06 (85/80). As you can see the index score equivalent here is quite different and doesn't take into account the end points (Optimal and Minimum expectancy levels).

PROGRAM EVALUATION MODELS (MATRIX)

Examples of program evaluation systems for comprehensive inpatient rehabilitation, subacute rehabilitation, and outpatient rehabilitation are shown in Appendices A–C. Each PE system has its own unique set of program objectives, recommended measures, who it is applied to, time of measure, data source, and expectancy levels. However, there may be similarities in the PE systems, particularly between comprehensive inpatient and subacute rehabilitation programs. The relative weights have been omitted from the models, because they tend to be different in each facility. The recommended measures tend to include both criteria (percent who reach a specified outcome by discharge) and improvement measures (average gain in FIM, self-care, mobility etc.), which are discussed in more detail in Chapter 10 on "Methods of Presenting and Reporting Outcome Results." ■

TABLE 2.
COMPREHENSIVE INPATIENT REHAB PROGRAM OBJECTIVES

INDEX SCORE	1	2	3	4	5	6	7	8	9	10	11	INDEX SCORE
Optimal 150	27.0	90%	1.60	18.0	1.60	2.10	90%	0.90	90%	90%	0.0%	Optimal 150
145	26.6	89%	1.57	18.3	1.58	2.07	89%	0.88	89%	89%	0.5%	145
140	26.2	88%	1.53	18.6	1.56	2.04	88%	0.86	88%	88%	1.0%	140
135	25.8	87%	1.50	18.9	1.54	2.01	87%	0.84	87%	87%	1.5%	135
130	25.4	86%	1.46	19.2	1.52	1.98	86%	0.82	86%	86%	2.0%	130
125	25.0	85%	1.43	19.5	1.50	1.95	85%	0.80	85%	85%	2.5%	125
120	24.6	84%	1.39	19.8	1.48	1.92	84%	0.78	84%	84%	3.0%	120
115	24.2	83%	1.36	20.1	1.46	1.89	83%	0.76	83%	83%	3.5%	115
110	23.8	82%	1.32	20.4	1.44	1.86	82%	0.74	82%	82%	4.0%	110
105	23.4	81%	1.29	20.7	1.42	1.83	81%	0.72	81%	81%	4.5%	105
Goal 100	23.0	80%	1.25	21.0	1.40	1.80	80%	0.70	80%	80%	5.0%	Goal 100
95	22.6	79%	1.22	21.3	1.38	1.77	79%	0.68	79%	79%	5.5%	95
90	22.2	78%	1.18	21.6	1.36	1.74	78%	0.66	78%	78%	6.0%	90
85	21.8	77%	1.15	21.9	1.34	1.71	77%	0.64	77%	77%	6.5%	85
80	21.4	76%	1.11	22.2	1.32	1.68	76%	0.62	76%	76%	7.0%	80
75	21.0	75%	1.08	22.5	1.30	1.65	75%	0.60	75%	75%	7.5%	75
70	20.6	74%	1.04	22.8	1.28	1.62	74%	0.58	74%	74%	8.0%	70
65	20.2	73%	1.01	23.1	1.26	1.59	73%	0.56	73%	73%	8.5%	65
60	19.8	72%	0.97	23.4	1.24	1.56	72%	0.54	72%	72%	9.0%	60
55	19.4	71%	0.94	23.7	1.22	1.53	71%	0.52	71%	71%	9.5%	55
Minimal 50	19.0	70%	0.90	24.0	1.20	1.50	70%	0.50	70%	70%	10.0%	Minimal 50

5. OVERVIEW OF QUALITY MANAGEMENT

WHAT IS QUALITY MANAGEMENT?

Quality management is an even broader concept than program evaluation and includes all aspects of the organization, including patient care. Quality management is the broadest of the three concepts and includes measures of performance in all major functions (both patient focused and organization functions) and is assessed in terms of the nine dimensions of quality.

Quality management is important in view of the changing emphasis of managed care entities. Provider organizations are reevaluating and changing their organizational structures, systems, and processes to gain further improvements in quality, outcome, and cost-effectiveness.

DEFINITION OF QUALITY

Quality can be defined as meeting or exceeding the customers' expectations. It is extremely important to identify the various customer groups and their outcome expectations, regardless of level of care, before developing a quality management system.

WHY IS QUALITY IMPROVEMENT IMPORTANT?

Although price is currently most important to payers, in the near future, payers will begin to demand outcome data, government will be asking for such data, and employers will be looking for value. The health care reform movement and development of provider report cards will eventually force providers to compare their results and share them with the general public.

A number of class action suits have recently been filed against the nation's largest managed care companies. The main issue focuses around denied access to reasonable and medically necessary services. Several of these cases have recently settled and are likely to force managed care entities to pay more attention to quality and outcome measures in addition to cost.

CHANGING EMPHASIS OF MANAGED CARE ENTITIES

The primary concern of most managed care companies today is cost of health care. Managed care companies tend to select providers solely on the basis of cost, whether it be a capitated rate (e.g., $1.10/member/month), a per diem (e.g., $450/day for subacute rehabilitation), or a discounted fee for service model (e.g., 25 percent below relative value units or reasonable and customary fees). Although they are interested in quality of care, it is assumed and expected from providers. Most managed care companies are not well informed about quality and outcome management. However, in the near future (within 12–18 months) managed care companies will begin to demand quality and outcome data from their contract providers, to protect them from any risk or liability exposure resulting from denial or restricted access to care.

Many managed care companies, workers' compensation carriers, and other third party payers are looking to accreditation standards such as those put out by CARF, JCAHO, and the Accreditation Council as criteria for selecting and contracting with providers.

The managed care companies will set up systems to continually monitor the quality, outcome, client satisfaction, and undesirable consequences of care for various providers. Senior citizens are enrolling in managed care plans and assigning their Medicare benefits to these plans in increasing numbers. Because the majority of occupational therapy services are provided to Medicare patients in most settings, providers are in a very tenuous position.

JCAHO'S SHIFT IN FOCUS

JCAHO is shifting its focus from process to outcomes, while at the same time incorporating some of the concepts of total quality management, performance improvement, and business practices into its description of quality management.

COPING WITH THE CHANGES

There is a short window of opportunity for occupational therapy providers to help define accreditation standards, develop quality and outcome measures, and design evaluation systems so they can influence what criteria are used by managed care entities, governmental agencies, and employers in evaluating providers. Providers should be prepared to address the outcome expectations of managed care entities: qualifications and expertise of providers, injury/re-injury prevention, medical complications, long-term outcomes, total case costs, and reduction of future health care usage.

ESSENTIAL ELEMENTS FOR QUALITY MANAGEMENT

In order to develop a quality management system, you must become familiar with:

- customer groups and some of their outcome expectations

- the JCAHO Standards for Improving Organizational Performance

- the Accreditation Council's outcome-based performance measures

- clinical benchmarking.

JCAHO has abandoned its 10-step model of quality management and now requires accredited organizations to develop a more comprehensive, systematic, organizationwide approach to performance improvement. Like CARF and the Accreditation Council, JCAHO standards only provide a framework and general requirements for how to approach a quality management program. Providers or facilities must comply with the standards of their accrediting agencies to remain fully accredited. Since the JCAHO criteria appear to be more encompassing, providers may find that they also may be able to satisfy the requirements of other organizations. JCAHO and CARF accreditation are tied to licensing and reimbursement in some states.

IMPLEMENTING QUALITY MANAGEMENT

The process of setting up a quality management system involves:

- identifying customer groups

- understanding customers' expectations

- determining whether to use the JCAHO or Accreditation Council model

- following the JCAHO or Accreditation Council guidelines

- using clinical benchmarking and clinical pathways.

IDENTIFYING CUSTOMER GROUPS (EXTERNAL AND INTERNAL)

Most occupational therapy providers tend to think of the patient, family and referring physician as their primary customers. However, providers frequently interact with other external customers, including attorneys, community physicians, employers, insurance case managers, managed care companies, government, licensing, and accreditation bodies. Table 3 provides a list of external and internal customer groups with whom an occupational therapy practitioner may interact. Each major and most influential customer group should be surveyed regarding its performance and outcome expectations of the occupational therapy provider before a quality management and outcome evaluation system is designed. The expectations of the internal customers inside the provider organization, clinic, or agency also should be considered. Often their expectations deal with efficiency, timeliness, accuracy, and productivity issues.

TABLE 3.
CUSTOMERS IDENTIFIED

External Customers	Internal Customers
Accreditation agencies	Administration
Attorneys	Admissions
Clients	Boards of director
Community physicians	Business office
Employers	Case management
Families	Data processing
Insurance case managers	Finance
Government agencies	Human resources
Managed care companies	Laboratory
The public	Medical records
Referring hospitals	Medical staff
Referring physicians	Nursing
Patients	Patient accounts
Professional organizations	Physical therapy
Peer review organization (PRO)	Psychology
Stockholders	Quality management
Third party payers	Social service
Vendors (durable medical equipment [DME] and suppliers)	Speech pathology

DETERMINING CUSTOMERS' OUTCOME EXPECTATIONS

You must know the customers' information needs and outcome expectations in order to collect and report the right type of quality and outcome information. Each customer group may have an entirely different set of outcome expectations of the occupational therapy provider. For example, insurance case managers and managed care companies have become increasingly concerned about the qualifications and expertise of providers, long-term outcomes, total case costs, and future health care use rates. The patient, on the other hand, may be hoping for a full functional recovery (e.g., total functional independence), which may be inconsistent with the payer's expectations. There needs to be a delicate balance between the patient's, family's, and payer's expectations, so that reasonable program/treatment goals can be established.

Studies have shown differences among various customers' expectations. Research on brain injury rehabilitation[210,212,215] indicated that the outcome expectations of payers, providers, and patients/families are not the same. In an effort to identify the most important outcome objectives for comprehensive outpatient rehabilitation centers/programs, a study conducted by the California Association of Rehabilitation Facilities and National Medical Enterprises in 1993[161] surveyed over 35 rehabilitation providers, experienced case managers, and third party payers who were knowledgeable about rehabilitation delivery systems. Respondents were asked to rate the relative importance (1 = not important, 10 = extremely important) of each of 10 outcome objectives that were initially perceived to be important for outpatient rehabilitation. Respondents were also given an opportunity to add and rate additional outcome objectives. The providers, who were mostly outpatient program managers, placed much more importance on customer satisfaction (i.e., patient, family, and referring physician) and maximization of functional independence and productivity. Payers, in contrast, were more concerned with prevention of injury/reinjury, medical complications, long-term outcomes, total case costs, and reduction of future health care usage. Payers also mentioned a number of other outcome issues that had more to do with expectations of the provider than with expected patient outcomes, such as: good communication with payer, good patient follow-up, treatment of the payer as a team member, honest (valid) outcome claims, and provision of what is medically reasonable and necessary. Similar results were obtained by the American Rehabilitation Association in an evaluation study of the RQI Network[217], and by the American Congress of Rehabilitation Medicine Head Injury ISIG[208] in 1994.

DETERMINING WHICH MODEL TO USE

The JCAHO approach to performance improvement[5] is an organizationwide approach that incorporates quality performance measures and expected outcomes along with the important organizational functions and quality dimensions. Although included, the patient is not necessarily the focal point of all performance improvement efforts. In contrast, the Accreditation Council[1] places the focus on client-centered outcome measures. Process variables are important only in the context of expected client outcomes. Individual decision making and choice are fundamental for outcomes to be achieved.

The JCAHO model is an organizationwide approach to performance improvement and therefore the most encompassing of the three models. However, an early child development or pediatric rehabilitation program may need to comply with the requirements from the Accreditation

Council. Some rehabilitation providers and facilities are solely accredited by CARF, but most have both CARF and JCAHO accreditation. Continued accreditation by these agencies may be a criterion for licensure and reimbursement in some states. An administrator should follow the guidelines and model from the appropriate accreditation organization.

USING THE JCAHO PERFORMANCE IMPROVEMENT MODEL

DEFINITION OF PERFORMANCE IMPROVEMENT.

In the 1996 *Accreditation Manual*[2,4], JCAHO describes *performance improvement* as a planned, systematic, and organizationwide approach to designing, measuring, assessing, and improving organizational performance. The approach involves collaboration and participation from all disciplines and levels of the organization.

The underlying assumptions are:

- The quality of service or product is determined by a careful understanding of the needs and expectations of customers.

- The organization's leaders have a responsibility for improving performance, acquiring the necessary knowledge, and setting priorities for performance improvement activities.

- The improvement of quality is continuous and never ending (CQI management philosophy).

- Everyone in the organization should be involved in improving quality.

UNDERSTANDING QUALITY PERFORMANCE DIMENSIONS

Quality performance dimensions are a set of fundamental elements for change. They provide the framework or blueprint around which quality improvement is planned, implemented, and evaluated. Nine dimensions of quality performance are identified in the 1996 JCAHO standards, as shown below.

JCAHO QUALITY PERFORMANCE DIMENSIONS

1. *Efficacy* of the procedure/treatment: The degree to which care of the patient has been shown to accomplish desired or projected outcomes.

2. *Appropriateness* of the test/procedure/service: The degree to which the care is relevant to the patient's clinical needs.

3. *Availability* of needed test/procedure/treatment/service: The degree to which appropriate care is available to meet the patient's needs.

4. *Timeliness* of test/procedure/treatment/service: The degree to which care is provided to the patient at the most beneficial or necessary time.

5. *Effectiveness* of test/procedures/treatments/services: The degree to which care is provided in the correct manner, given the current state of knowledge, to achieve the desired or projected outcomes.

6. *Continuity* of services/practitioners and providers: The degree to which care is coordinated and consistent among practitioners or organizations over time.

7. *Safety:* The degree to which intervention and environmental risks are minimized for the patient and others, including the health care provider.

8. *Efficiency:* The relationship between outcomes (results of treatment) and the resources used to deliver patient care.

9. *Respect and caring:* The degree to which the patient or a designee is involved in his or her own care decisions, and the degree to which those providing services are sensitive to and respect the patient's needs, expectations, and individual preferences.

DETERMINING WHICH FUNCTIONS TO ASSESS

Under the 1996 JCAHO standards a number of important organizational functions, which may vary according to practice setting, should be assessed in terms of the appropriate dimensions of quality performance:

PATIENT-FOCUSED FUNCTIONS

- patient rights and organizational ethics
- assessment of patients
- care of patients
- education
- continuum of care

ORGANIZATION FUNCTIONS

- improvement organizational performance
- leadership
- management of the care environment
- management of human resources
- management of information
- surveillance, prevention, and control of infections.

SELECTING PERFORMANCE MEASURES

Appropriate indicators and performance measures should be established for each organizational function and quality dimension. The criteria for selecting performance measures should include:

- assessment of the dimensions of quality performance relevant to the important functions of the organization
- measures of both processes and outcomes

- a comprehensive set of performance measures for both priority areas and continuing measurement of stability of important processes (indicators)

- high-risk, high-volume, and/or problem-prone processes

- other sensors of performance: needs, expectations and feedback of patients and others (customer satisfaction), results of ongoing activities designed to control infections, safety, or care environment

- staff views regarding current performance and opportunities for improvement.

ANALYZING THE RESULTS

Based on objective measurement of performance of existing processes, outcomes of care, and major functions, the organization should be able to analyze and interpret the results to determine:

- whether design specifications of new process of care were met

- the current level of performance and stability of current processes of care

- priorities for areas that can be improved

- actions required to improve performance

- effectiveness of implemented strategies to improve performance.

ESTABLISHING THRESHOLD VALUES

The pertinent quality performance questions should be clearly identified prior to collecting and analyzing the data. The data should be analyzed against predetermined performance expectations (thresholds), design specifications, or other applicable performance improvement criteria. Appropriate threshold values should be established for each indicator for all important functions and dimensions of care, based on:

- internal processes and outcomes over time (trends)

- comparisons to relevant scientific, clinical, and management literature; practice guidelines or parameters; and clinical pathways

- comparison to external reference groups and databases as appropriate

- comparison to best practices or benchmarks, when appropriate.

Should the analysis of results indicate a significant or undesirable variation from expected performance, then a more intensified assessment (focused study) should be initiated to determine possible causes and possible solutions for the variance. Caution should be exercised when comparing results to external reference groups and databases to ensure the data are severity adjusted before any final conclusions have been reached.

ACCREDITATION COUNCIL MODEL

Although there are some similarities to the JCAHO model in terms of important organizational functions, all aspects of quality and outcome in the Accreditation Council's model relate to the client.

According to the Accreditation Council, outcome-based performance measures should fall into the following dimensions:

- personal goals

- choice

- social inclusion

- relationships

- rights

- dignity and respect

- health

- environment

- security

- satisfaction.

CLINICAL BENCHMARKING

The goals of clinical benchmarking are to create a sense of what is achievable and to find out ways of achieving it. This involves gaining insight into how superior results are produced, and studying how specific processes of care are applied to specific diagnoses. Randomized clinical trials can be helpful to isolate important determinants and prognostic indicators for positive outcomes. The occupational therapy practitioner should try to gain insight into what factors (i.e., client, clinical, treatment techniques, and other environmental factors) tend to lead to the best results. The best place to start is to review the success cases and determine what is unique or different about those clients and how they were treated. Clinical benchmarking involves research to identify the best practices and parameters that have been demonstrated to produce the best possible results with the least amount of variation for a given diagnostic or impairment group and specialty. Practice parameters are agreed upon strategies for patient management that are within the range of acceptable practice established by a professional organization. One must identify the benchmark facilities and programs and establish a target for clinical performance based on best practices and comparisons to like providers.

Clinical pathways (critical pathways) should be developed based on the expected outcome, progress and recovery pattern, functional status, treatment interventions, tests/procedures/services, and other resources required to ensure the best possible outcome with the least amount of variation. The clinical pathways become the standard road map for decision making at each stage of recovery and treatment, and should transcend the entire continuum of care for a particular disability or impairment. Through clinical pathways and effective case management systems, providers can increase the likelihood (predictability) of desired or positive outcome results. ∎

III.
GENERAL ISSUES, TECHNIQUES, AND PROCEDURES FOR OUTCOME EVALUATION

6. KEY SUCCESS FACTORS

Some of the continuous quality improvement strategies that have proven to be most effective for rehabilitation providers, including occupational therapy practitioners, are as follows:

- involving staff

- studying the clinical outcome data available

- making comparisons to external reference groups or databases

- improving outcome data management

- providing training on how to effectively use outcome evaluation to improve performance

- producing narrative executive summaries

- evaluating the clinical processes of care for specific diagnoses

- gaining insight into how to produce superior results

- identifying the benchmark facilities and programs

- developing clinical (critical) pathways that are outcome oriented

- developing effective case management

- reengineering the delivery process to ensure that the best possible outcomes are achieved at the lowest possible cost.

Each of these strategies are discussed briefly in the following section.

INVOLVING STAFF

The single most common reason for failure of evaluation efforts is the lack of staff involvement in the development and implementation of the system.[103,187,192] Direct involvement of staff is both prudent and necessary. Staff must have a commitment to the evaluation system because they are the ones responsible for providing the services and for supplying much of the data. Staff participation can greatly increase the technical quality of the evaluation system. Furthermore, staff can contribute to setting realistic expectations of program outcomes and goals. Results are then much more meaningful to staff, and more likely to enhance morale, initiative, and cooperation.

Staff often fear that an evaluation system will not adequately measure the quality and outcome of services provided. A typical comment about functional assessment is that the instruments are not sensitive to small increments of improvement and do not show patient progress.

Therefore, staff should be involved in developing the outcome evaluation system and measures. Staff participation in evaluation system development may appear time consuming and costly. When viewed from the perspective of technical soundness and the need for proper installation and maintenance of the evaluation system, staff involvement during development will likely reduce the long-term cost of the system.

STUDYING CLINICAL OUTCOME DATA

It is important for the evaluation and program manager to first study the clinical outcome data and become familiar with the measurement scales, sensitivity, reliability, validity, discriminative power, and predictive ability in terms of other performance measures and handicap issues. Comparisons should be made to external reference groups, databases, practice parameters, guidelines, and published scientific results for various treatment strategies and settings. The evaluator should then attempt to identify the potential clinical, practice, program, financial, operational, and client outcome implications of the data and results.

IMPROVING OUTCOME DATA MANAGEMENT

Sometimes the answers may lie in better outcome data management. Important tasks for improving outcome data management include:

- establishing the accuracy and appropriateness of clinical and client assessments and ratings

- ensuring accurate coding of data

- conducting error checks for missing or inconsistent information

- ensuring timeliness of assessments

- establishing client self-report measures and compliance

- determining the availability of required data

- standardizing reporting

- conducting appropriate statistical analysis of data.

The ability to interface or integrate various clinical, outcome, financial, and billing systems may eliminate unnecessary duplicate entries and improve the accuracy of data recorded.

PROVIDING TRAINING ON HOW TO USE OUTCOME EVALUATION TO IMPROVE PERFORMANCE

Unfortunately, most clinicians do not instinctively know how to use outcome results to improve program performance. They may not have training in evaluation research and may have difficulty interpreting the results and identifying the potential clinical, operational, and practice implications. Training must be provided for clinical, medical, and management staff on how to effectively use outcome evaluation to improve performance. A number of good textbooks and seminars are available that can provide background information and strategies. However, the training usually has to be customized to the particular practice setting and program emphasis.

PRODUCING EXECUTIVE SUMMARIES OF RESULTS

Clinical and management staff often do not have the time or interest to sift through volumes of outcome results, reports, and statistics. An executive summary can be useful to highlight certain important findings, provide an interpretation of the results, and identify program strengths and opportunities for performance improvement. An executive summary also can suggest strategies for improving quality, outcome results, cost-effectiveness, and client satisfaction, as well as suggesting areas where more intensified studies may be appropriate.

EVALUATING THE CLINICAL PROCESSES OF CARE

The clinical team and occupational therapy practitioner need to carefully evaluate the clinical processes and critical aspects of care for each diagnosis or impairment group treated in the program. Randomized clinical trails can be helpful here to isolate important determinants and prognostic indicators for positive outcomes.

GAINING INSIGHT INTO PRODUCING SUPERIOR RESULTS

The occupational therapy practitioner should try to gain insight into what factors (i.e., client, clinic, treatment techniques, procedures, intervention strategies, diagnostic tests/evaluations, family and support systems, and other environmental factors) tend to lead to the best results. The best place to start is to review the success cases and determine what was unique or different about those clients and how they were treated.

IDENTIFYING THE BENCHMARK FACILITIES AND PROGRAMS

Providers need to identify the benchmark facilities and programs, find out their trade secrets, and attempt to emulate or duplicate their successful program strategies. This usually is easier to accomplish within a closed system of providers who may be more willing to share their success strategies. Providers who participate in an external reference group or data management service often seek to protect the anonymity and confidentiality of their program and client results. Some may be reluctant to share their trade secrets initially, but government and managed care entities eventually will exert pressure on those providers to disclose and publish their best practices.

DEVELOPING CLINICAL (CRITICAL) PATHWAYS

Most occupational therapy practitioners have been involved to some extent in development of critical pathways, which are process and procedure oriented, and in mapping out a treatment regime for a given diagnosis or impairment. Clinical pathways are systematic, interdisciplinary outcome-oriented tools. They identify key aspects of care that are critical to ensuring optimum patient outcome and map them along a timeline that usually covers the full continuum of care (all practice settings). Clinical pathways, therefore, need to include process, recovery, and expected outcome elements. The objectives of clinical pathways are to understand and improve the processes of care, rationalize care, minimize unexpected or undesirable variance, and standardize clinical practice to enhance the predictability of positive or best possible outcomes.

DEVELOPING AN EFFECTIVE CASE MANAGEMENT SYSTEM

A well-developed case management system is essential to monitor patient progress toward expected outcomes, resource use, and efficient and effective transitions across the continuum of care. Outcome measures may assist in the initial level of care decisions, type and intensity of services required, and the decision to transition a patient to the next level of care or practice setting. The goal of rehabilitation has shifted to "optimizing functional recovery" and transitioning the patient, as soon as it is safe to do so, to the least costly setting, thereby maximizing cost-effectiveness across the entire continuum of care. This requires real-time interaction with clinical, progress, and outcome results on a frequent basis (often daily or weekly) to ensure that the patient is still on track with the clinical pathway and expected outcome. Providers must have an effective case management system to survive under a capitated health care system. The risk of efficient and effective clinical resource management will be shifted to the providers. ■

7. CONSIDERATIONS IN CHOOSING AN OUTCOME MEASURE

Occupational therapists in all practice settings are looking for appropriate outcome measures for clinical, research, program evaluation, management, and marketing purposes. The tendency of most therapists is to look for a single outcome measure that is capable of meeting multiple needs and applications. Often, occupational therapy practitioners tend to gravitate toward refined measures of *performance components* such as sensory, motor, perceptual, or neuromuscular function rather than focus on general outcome measures of *performance areas*. The following section explains some key factors that should be considered in choosing or designing outcome measures:

- goals and objectives of the program

- impairment groups to be evaluated

- global versus impairment-specific measures

- time frames in which measures will be applied

- accuracy and precision of results (i.e., validity, reliability, measurement and scaling properties, and sensitivity)

- expertise and time required to complete the assessment

- continuity of measures across time and settings

- integration with existing documentation and management information systems (MIS)

- comparison with other providers.

CLARIFYING THE GOALS AND OBJECTIVES OF THE PROGRAM

The first step in determining the appropriate outcome measure is to clearly state the goals and objectives of the program or service. The outcome objectives will vary by program, population served, and customer. It is extremely important to identify the customer's expectations at this point. The program goals and objectives should be consistent with the mission and philosophy of the organization and include input from the patients, families, care practitioners, referring physicians, third party payers, and other major customer groups. The focus of most outpatient programs seems to be more on handicap measures and added value, rather than just functional restoration, pain reduction, strength, and endurance.

EXAMPLE OF GOALS FOR A WORK-HARDENING PROGRAM

The goals of a work-hardening program for injured workers with the potential for returning to work and productive activities might include:

- maximize functional independence

- increase psychosocial adjustment

- increase functional work capacity

- prevent reinjury

- improve the use of proper body mechanics

- decrease subjective pain

- minimize duration of treatment

- maximize customer satisfaction

- return to gainful employment/productive activities.

This is accomplished through a comprehensive, interdisciplinary, and individualized treatment program that incorporates real or simulated work tasks. The program is designed to minimize risk and optimize work capabilities of persons served.

DETERMINING WHICH IMPAIRMENT GROUPS TO EVALUATE

It is essential to identify the caseload composition, impairments, and diagnostic groups to be evaluated before selecting outcome measures. An outcome measure may be appropriate for one group and not for others.

GLOBAL VERSUS IMPAIRMENT-SPECIFIC MEASURES

Global cross-sectional outcome measures such as the FIM^{SM}, LORS, RESTORE, and PECS (all of which are defined in Chapter 8) may provide some general clinical and functional outcomes across many impairment groups, but may not be sensitive to the unique clinical aspects for a specific impairment group (i.e., brain injury). The outcome measure also should be sensitive to small increments of improvement and process that may vary by impairment group. **There is no one single measure that is appropriate for all impairment groups and practice settings.** Still, many providers tend to look for a "gold standard" single measure system, and they become frustrated with the instruments when they attempt to apply them to different populations and settings. They also may gravitate toward refined measures of *performance components* such as sensory, motor, perceptual, or neuromuscular function rather than focusing on general outcome measures or *performance areas*. A combination of global outcome measures and impairment-specific measures usually is recommended.

DECIDING WHEN TO MEASURE OUTCOMES

Time of application of measure may be critical in deciding which measure to use. Outcomes should be measured when the results are most stable and reflective of treatment/program interventions. Generally outcomes should be measured at discharge and 6 to 12 months after termination of services depending on the focus of the program and the populations served. After termination of outpatient services, handicap measures of societal disadvantage, customer satisfaction, return to work or productive lifestyle, perception of wellness, and future health care use are more appropriate than measures of impairment or disability.

COLLECTING FOLLOW-UP INFORMATION

It is difficult and often costly for many providers to perform follow-up evaluation. The three methods most commonly used to collect follow-up information[120] are:

1. follow-up return visit or reevaluation

2. mailed follow-up survey

3. telephone interview.

Some providers use a combination of all three to capture patient follow-up information.

Follow-Up Visit. The follow-up return visit involves scheduling and bringing the patient back into the facility or clinic for a reevaluation. If assessment is done during a routine medical follow-up visit, it may be easier to obtain the outcome data and get reimbursed for the assessment. Unfortunately, not all patients are available for follow-up visits, and the cancellation or no-show rates may run as high as 40 percent.

Mailed Survey. Facilities that use the mailed follow-up survey often find that there is little control over accuracy of information and the return rates tend to be low (20–30 percent of questionnaires mailed out). There are a few methods for enhancing the response rates, but they require additional time, energy, and money. Most experts agree that response rates under 40 percent (depending on number of patients served) can present problems of sampling bias. Because mailed questionnaires often are completed by the patient, family member, or significant other, they may be subject to certain response sets (the tendency to respond to questions in predictable ways). Attitudes, emotional reaction or strain, fatigue, pain, fluctuations in attention or coordination, family problems, and financial problems can influence the way a person may respond to the questions at a given point in time.

Telephone Interview. Facilities also may choose to collect follow-up information through a structured telephone interview. The interview itself should be brief, well structured, and limited to no more than 20–30 minutes.[120] The use of standard protocols of probe questions and decision trees can greatly streamline the telephone interview and improve the accuracy of information obtained. Paraprofessionals, college student, OT interns, and volunteers can be used to obtain follow-up information over the telephone more cost effectively.[86] Occasionally, responses obtained from the patient, family member, and significant others should be compared with results obtained during a follow-up return visit (see inter-informant and inter-procedural reliability in this section under the heading of reliability).

ENSURING ACCURACY AND PRECISION OF RESULTS

The accuracy and precision of results must meet acceptable measurement standards.[133] An error in assessing functional abilities, limitations, or medical status could lead to a false conclusion that patients have deteriorated when they have actually improved or at least maintained their gain in functional abilities (performance areas) from occupational therapy. Each outcome measure chosen must have adequate validity, reliability, and demonstrated measurement properties, sufficient sensitivity to measure small increments of improvement or change, and the ability to discriminate among various patient populations.

VALIDITY

Validity is a critical factor to consider when choosing an outcome measure. Validity refers to the extent to which the test measures what it is intended to measure. How appropriate, meaningful, and useful is a measure and the inferences made from it? There are five types of validity.

1. *Criteria-referenced validity* is the extent to which a test score predicts an outcome or correlates with other information currently available that is external to the measure. For example, an occupational therapist working with a child with learning disabilities might want to know how well the child is able to function in the classroom and at home (performance contexts), but the therapist cannot conduct extended observations and evaluations in these settings. The practitioner, therefore might use tests of sensory/ motor/perceptual skills, along with feedback from parents and teachers, as a proxy for how well the child is likely to perform in these settings.

2. *Concurrent validity.* In the preceding example, the degree to which the measures reflect actual home/classroom functioning is an issue of concurrent validity. Another application of concurrent validity is the correlation with other similar outcome measures.

3. *Predictive validity* is the extent to which a measure is able to forecast some future event. For example, the SF-36[95], a widely used measure of patient perception of wellness, has been used to predict future health care use among patients with cardiac, pulmonary, infectious disease, and medically complex conditions. The impact of occupational therapy treatment intervention on future health care use rates may have multiple determining factors. Multiple measures often are needed to fully understand the outcomes and predict future events. Craig Velozo, in an article in the October 1994 issue of the *American Journal of Occupational Therapy* (AJOT)[101], argued that the choice of a single outcome measure (or gold standard) may compromise sensitivity to true functional outcomes obtained by OT and limit the ability to predict future healthcare costs and savings.

4. *Construct validity* is the degree to which an instrument measures the theoretical construct it was designed to measure. Establishing adequate construct validity requires piecing together a network of relationships. Determining whether a measure distinguishes among impairment groups, levels of severity, discharge disposition, resource utilization, return to work, or productive activities are examples of construct validity.

5. *Content validity* is concerned with the extent to which measures represent all facets of the factor or behavior being assessed. If the test measures independence in self-care (ADL), then all major items in that domain should be sampled. Factor analysis, item analysis and *Rasch analysis* can be used to assess the measurement properties, scaling, and grouping of items in an inventory. *Factor analysis* is a method of analyzing relationships (correlations) among many variables, grouping the items into common factors, and simplifying the measure. An *item analysis* measures how well each item predicts the total score or subscores for high- and low-functioning patients and different impairment groups. The Rasch analysis provides evidence of the scaling properties, precision, unidimensionality, item weighting, and fit of the items within a category or inventory. Rasch analysis can transform ratings on an ordinal scale to an interval scale equivalent for applications of appropriate parametric statistics. Most outcome measures in occupational therapy practice settings are ordinal scales. It is necessary to use Rasch analysis to verify the scaling properties, unidimensionality, item weighting, and fit, and to transform the scale into an interval equivalent so evaluators can apply appropriate parametric statistics such as gain scores, standard deviations, and means to test the significance of functional improvements. Otherwise the evaluator may be led to making false conclusions about the results. As mentioned by Craig Velozo[101], a Rasch analysis of the FIM[SM], LORS, and PECS demonstrated that all three instruments measured similar domains of performance with varying degrees of precision. The FIM[SM] and LORS tended to have ceiling effects (maximum obtainable outcome) with certain types of patients that may limit their suitability for postacute and outpatient settings.

RELIABILITY

Reliability is the extent to which ratings on an instrument are consistent and reproducible when administered under similar circumstances. There are three basic types of reliability.

1. *Test–retest reliability,* or stability over time, is the degree to which scores remain the same upon retesting, all other factors being constant. In most occupational practice settings, it is difficult to measure this type of reliability because patients change over time. The time interval between repeated measures must be short, while avoiding any practice effect.

2. *Interrater reliability* is the degree to which measures are applied in the same way by different observers. The outcome measure must have adequate interrater reliability (r2 > .85, or a Kappa Coefficient > .75, depending on size of sample). Training, video tapes, educational materials, and credentialing or certifying raters can help enhance interrater agreement. In addition, one should also evaluate *interdisciplinary reliability* (between different disciplines), *interprocedural reliability* (differences between results from personal observations, telephone interview, or mailed follow-up survey), and *interinformant reliability* (differences between patient, caregiver, spouse, or significant other).

3. *Internal consistency* means that all the items of a test are intercorrelated so that the trait being measured is measured by all items. The unidimensionality (same domain) of a scale is equally important. Here both factor analysis and Rasch analysis can help shed

some light on the properties of the instruments, discriminative power, and grouping of items.

SENSITIVITY

The outcome tool needs to be sensitive enough to measure the small increments of change that are likely to be the product of occupational therapy efforts. Outcome measures need to reflect change or improvement in function. The primary criticism of the FIM[SM] is that it is not sensitive to change in the outpatient rehabilitation populations; patients reach their maximum functioning level very quickly and have limited ability to show further gains on the scale. The outcome measure also needs to be sensitive to temporal and environmental aspects (performance contexts).

DETERMINING THE EXPERTISE AND TIME REQUIRED

Some measures require the specialized expertise of a specific discipline and training to complete the assessment, while other outcome measures can be completed by any trained clinician. Time to complete the assessment is another important consideration. Functional assessments should not be cumbersome for staff to complete. Some of the outcome measures like the PECS, RIC-FAS III, and APGs may take over an hour to complete while others can be completed in fewer than 30 minutes. The use of simple checklist, coding systems, and abstracts can greatly simplify data collection.

ENSURING CONTINUITY OF MEASURES ACROSS SETTINGS

Is the outcome tool appropriate to measure performance over time? In an attempt to select a measure that is appropriate for tracking patient progress over a longer period of time (e.g., 1–2 years), one sacrifices sensitivity to small changes that may occur during a shorter time period (e.g., 1–3 months). Consideration also must be given to outcome measures that may be suitable for multiple practice settings across the continuum of care. This is particularly important when the same clinicians are rendering treatment in multiple care settings. Formations in Health Care[87] has taken a lead in attempting to define and measure outcomes across the continuum of care. There may be some common data elements and inventory items that are appropriate to use in all practice settings, but it is unlikely that one outcome measure will be suitable and sufficient for all settings.

INTEGRATING WITH EXISTING DOCUMENTATION MIS

Before implementing an outcome evaluation system for a particular program or practice setting, one should carefully assess the potential impact on the organization in terms of costs, additional reporting requirements, the ability to interface with existing documentation, reporting requirements, and management information systems (MIS). The goal should be to streamline data collection, eliminate duplicative data entry, control accuracy and integrity of data from multiple sources, and provide timely and relevant data from program management and clinical decisions. A well-designed outcome evaluation system also may assist in automating clinical documentation, progress notes, and reports.

INTEGRATING WITH MIS

Outcome evaluation should be integrated with other management information systems such as financial systems, clinical/documentation systems, human resource systems, productivity and acuity systems, and marketing and planning systems, so that a provider and management team can look at all the variables to determine what contributes to the best possible outcome with the least amount of resource consumption.

Outcome evaluation also should be integrated with MIS reports such as productivity studies and revenue statistics, and staffing, census, and budget reports. When these types of feedback data are effectively integrated, it is possible to project growth rates for the program. As shown in Figure 9, outcome, billing, cost allocation, medical record, case mix, and census data can be integrated into one information system to produce management reports, planning reports, marketing reports, financial reports, and special studies. Data integration can reduce the overall reporting costs. Staffing, budgeting, equipment acquisitions, treatment techniques, and operating procedures can be modified to serve current and anticipated needs of clients.

FIGURE 9.

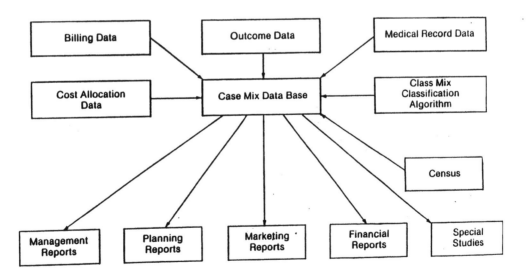

FACTORS TO CONSIDER

The extent to which different reporting systems can be integrated into a single system is a complex issue. The following factors must be considered when developing an integrated system:

- duplicate information

- control and integration of data from multiple sources

- timing requirements

- external approval from funding and regulatory agencies to modify source documents

- computer limitations and costs

- types of reports that are likely to be useful

- availability of data required.

INTEGRATION WITH QUALITY IMPROVEMENT SYSTEMS

Outcome evaluation reports can provide a more specific direction for quality improvement (QI) efforts and intensified QI studies. Management reports based on the outcome data may prompt individual chart audits and special studies to further assist in problem resolution. Outcome evaluation can provide an overall picture of performance and outcome[188], but it simply identifies problems and does not provide specific solutions. Special studies and intensified reviews are necessary to identify potential causes and solutions. According to the 1995 JCAHO standards[2], an intensified assessment should be conducted when an undesirable variation in outcome or performance measures has occurred. Organizations or providers may initiate an intensified assessment when they believe they can improve already good performance. The intensive assessment should be initiated based on important single events, undesirable levels, patterns, or trends. Appropriate statistical analyses should be used to identify possible causes.

COMPARISON WITH OTHER PROVIDERS

Many management decisions require the availability of comparative data from other similar providers. Certainly, JCAHO is encouraging providers to compare their results with external reference groups and participate in a data management service to obtain comparative data from other providers. Care must be taken, however, to ensure the data are severity adjusted to accommodate differences in case mix, severity of disabilities, medical acuity, and types of patients treated. What outcome measures are being used or under development by other providers? Other than those data management services mentioned here, is there a database or data management service that a provider can participate in and compare results to other similar providers? Providers' objectives should be to research what is available currently before attempting to develop their own outcome measures and evaluation systems.

USING DATA MANAGEMENT SERVICES

A data bank or common repository is needed to store and consolidate information supplied by individual facilities. A data management service can provide:

- a collection of primary data for user facilities on standardized formats

- verification of accuracy of data and quality control

- automated and computerized data analysis

- report generation for user facilities

- aggregate reporting of results from all user facilities

- data storage for future retrieval and analysis

- special studies for research purposes.

Several companies currently provide various types of data management services to rehabilitation providers. Some of these are shown below.

EXAMPLES OF DATA MANAGEMENT COMPANIES

Hospital Utilization Project (HUP)[48,50]

LORS American Data System (LADS, which is part of Formations in Health Care) [51,53]

Patient Evaluation Conference System (PECS)[46]

Shared Medical Systems (SMS)

National Easter Seal Society Data Management Service[54]

R/COM[55]

Data Med Clinical Support Services[42]

UE Net for Hand Therapy[56]

Uniform Data System for Medical Rehabilitation (UDS$_{MR}$^{SM}). [43,44,45]

The majority of these services is designed for medical rehabilitation, but some also may have application to other settings. Formations in Health Care also has developed the RESTORE[167] program for comprehensive outpatient programs, and has recently developed the Medical Outcome System (MOS)[52] for respiratory, pain, and wound subacute patients. According to their latest brochure they are also working on outcome systems for home health, occupational rehabilitation, and acute care. The Focus on Therapeutic Outcomes (FOTO, Inc.)[160], a consortium of outpatient rehabilitation providers, has developed an outcome database to measure and compare the functional outcomes of outpatient programs (primarily physical therapy) using a modified version of the SF-36 (discussed in Chapter 8) and selected demographic data for back, neck, knee, arthritis, pain, and orthopedic patients. UDS$_{MR}$^{SM} has established a separate SNF/Rehabilitation database[242] using the FIM^{SM} with over 100 subacute rehabilitation providers. Data Med[42] recently has developed an integrated software produce that incorporates both the Minimum Data Set (MDS) required in SNF and the FIM^{SM} for patient care planning and outcome.

COSTS

The cost of participating in these data services varies. An initial fee and annual fee usually are assessed plus a charge per abstract submitted for data processing. Total subscription costs range from $2,700/year to $7,500/year, depending on the size of the program, database, and reporting requirements.

JCAHO has been developing its own national indicator-based performance system called the Indicator Measurement System (IMSystem).[49] JCAHO will require all accredited agencies and providers to participate in an external data management service and reference group, and compare results with other cohort providers by 1997. ■

8. OUTCOME MEASURES AND SYSTEMS FOR INPATIENT AND HOSPITAL-BASED SETTINGS

Numerous outcome measures and systems are available and others currently are under development for a variety of occupational therapy practice settings and programs. This section covers outcome measures that can be used in inpatient and hospital-based settings, including comprehensive inpatient rehabilitation, subacute rehabilitation, and subacute medical, spinal cord injury, and brain injury programs. This is not an all-inclusive list but a description of commonly used instruments that meet most of the selection and measurement criteria mentioned in Chapter 7. For more detailed information on outcome measures for specific settings, programs, and impairment groups, see the reference list at the end of this guide in which references are listed by major category.

COMPREHENSIVE INPATIENT REHABILITATION

Outcome evaluation in comprehensive inpatient rehabilitation generally includes measures of medical outcomes, clinical outcomes (including functional status), and client satisfaction. Evaluators in the field of rehabilitation constantly are searching for objective, sensitive, and reliable functional assessment instruments. It is important to describe the functional level of patients when they enter a program, the amount of functional gains they made while in the program and after discharge, and the final functional outcome attained by patients at follow-up. Some of the common functional status measures are the Functional Independence Measure[SM] (FIM), LORS III American Data System (LADS), Patient Evaluation Conference System (PECS), the Rehabilitation Institute of Chicago—Functional Assessment Scale Version III (RIC-FAS III), and the Functional Assessment Measure (FAM).

USING FUNCTIONAL STATUS RATING INSTRUMENTS

Outcome evaluation in rehabilitation generally includes measures of medical and clinical outcomes, including functional status and client satisfaction. Evaluators in the field of rehabilitation are continually in search of objective, sensitive, and reliable functional assessment instruments. It is important to describe the functional level of patients upon entry into a program, the amount of functional gain made while in the program as well as after discharge, and the final functional outcome attained by patients at follow-up. Generally, this information is obtained using a functional status rating instrument to assess a patient's functional competency and independence in such areas as ADL, mobility, communication, psychosocial adjustment, cognitive functioning, and vocational adjustment. Rating scales assessing the degree of independence have ranged from a 3- to a 100-point scale. In most cases, an assessment of the level of independence takes into account the amount of assistance required to complete the activity, which is a measure of severity of disability or burden of care. The amount of assistance can easily be specified and operationally defined. The 3-point scales, such as the Barthel Index[33] and Katz Index of Independence[31], tend to divide performance as follows:

- unable to do the activity

- can complete the activity with help or assistive devices

- can complete the activity independently.

Several instruments[24,36,38], also take into consideration whether special equipment or preparation is needed. One rating instrument[24] also assesses the speed and overall efficiency with which the patient is able to complete the activity. Some rating instruments like the FIM[SM] yield a total or composite score for all the items in the inventory, while others provide subscores in each major category or domain such as self-care, mobility, or communication.

CHOOSING A FUNCTIONAL ASSESSMENT INSTRUMENT

When selecting a functional assessment instrument, the evaluator should remember that the instrument is intended to be an evaluation tool to assess global outcome and functioning, not a refined clinical instrument. Occupational therapy practitioners may tend to gravitate toward refined measures of *performance components* such as sensory, motor, perceptual, or neuro-muscular function rather than focusing on general *performance areas (outcomes)*. The outcome measures also should assess actual observed or practiced performance and behavior, rather than capacity.

FUNCTIONAL INDEPENDENCE MEASURE (FIM)

The FIM[SM] has become the most widely used and accepted measure of functional status in inpatient rehabilitation settings. The FIM is part of the Uniform Data System for Medical Rehabilitation (UDS$_{MR}$)[39], which collects data on 22 variables (demographic, outcome, length of stay, impairment grouping, charges, and follow-up information). There are currently over 800 UDS$_{MR}$[SM] subscribers, 687 of whom are enrolled as comprehensive medical rehabilitation facilities (203 free-standing rehabilitation hospitals and 484 acute rehabilitation units). As of December 31, 1994, 420 of these facilities were fully credentialed and reporting data to UDS$_{MR}$[SM] in Buffalo, NY. The FIM[SM] contains 18 items, rated on a 7-point scale, that measure level of independence and functional outcome. Ratings are established within 72 hours of admission and of discharge, and 80 to 180 days postdischarge from inpatient rehabilitation. The FIM[SM] is a measure of performance, not capacity, and was designed to be discipline free. The FIM[SM] was designed primarily for inpatient acute rehabilitation populations and follow-up, but may also be appropriate for subacute rehabilitation and some home health programs as well. UDS$_{MR}$[SM] currently is aggregating over 200,000 records annually. There were over 700,000 records in the database as of December 31, 1994.

UDS$_{MR}$[SM] has produced for and distributed to all subscribers a *Guide for the Uniform Data Set* version 4.0 (available in 8 languages)[39], training materials and videotapes, and a software product, FIMware™. The new FIMware™ allows facilities to aggregate their own data, graph results, and submit quarterly data to UDS$_{MR}$^{SM} and includes the FRG-Penn Stimulation Model. FIMware^{TM} also can export to other Windows-based applications such as Lotus, DBase, Excel, and Harvard Graphics so facilities can prepare their own reports. The FRG simulation model can be used to help establish appropriate LOS targets and FIM^{SM} discharge goals based on patient acuity, age, FIM^{SM} score at admittance, and impairment code. UDS$_{MR}$^{SM} provides each subscribing facility with quarterly and annual reports, and with regional, national, and statewide comparisons. The average cost of participation in UDS$_{MR}$^{SM} is $2,700/year: $1,700 for quarterly and annual reports, plus $32 per licensed and staffed bed for data processing (inpatient and follow-up data).

Credentialing Process. There is a two-phase credentialing process to ensure maximum reliability of the FIM^{SM} ratings and accurate and complete submission of UDS$_{MR}$^{SM} facility data. Phase I involves training and credentialing of all clinical staff in the use of the FIM^{SM} (interrater reliability). Phase II involves a technical review of two quarters worth of facility data for errors or incomplete records, coding inconsistencies, and significant variations from the profile of other providers. UDS$_{MR}$^{SM} provides regional training seminars on the FIM^{SM} in collaboration with the American Rehabilitation Association's Rehabilitation Research and Education Fund.

Aside from the credentialing process, considerable effort has been devoted to establishing the reliability and validity of the FIM^{SM}. According to UDS$_{MR}$^{SM}, the interrater reliability of subscriber facilities (fully credentialed) was 0.99 (r) for total FIM^{SM} score and a Kappa Coefficient of 0.66–0.83 for individual FIM^{SM} items. The reliability and validity of the FIM^{SM} have been well documented, and a Rasch analysis has provided further evidence of the scaling properties, precision, unidimensionality, weighting and fit of the FIM^{SM} items into two factors, Motor FIM^{SM} (items A–M) and Cognitive FIM^{SM} (items N–R). There are other pending studies of interdisciplinary reliability, interprocedural reliability (telephone vs. personal observation), interinformant (patient vs. significant other), and test–retest reliability. For more information contact UDS$_{MR}$^{SM} at (716) 289-2076 or write to: Uniform Data Systems for Medical Rehabilitation, 232 Parker Hall, State University of New York at Buffalo, 3435 Main St., Buffalo, NY 14214-3007.

LORS III AMERICAN DATA SYSTEM (LADS)

The LORS III American Data System (LADS)[51] is part of Formations in Health Care, Inc. Outcome Systems. There are currently 177 subscribers, 75 in the Acute Rehabilitation database. The LADS contains 32 indicators and includes facility descriptors, patient demographics, and functional assessment in ADL, mobility, verbal communication, written communication, alternative communication, cognitive ability, and short- and long-term memory. There also is an assessment of patient vocational status and satisfaction at follow-up. Functional status is established within 3 days of admission, 3 days of program completion, and 90 days after discharge from comprehensive inpatient rehabilitation. The rating scale, which is similar to the FIM^{SM}, is based on a 5-point scale (total assistance, maximum assistance, moderate assistance, minimal to standby assistance, and independent) with an option for no therapy planned/provided. A similar 5-point scale is provided for the communication, cognitive, and memory items. Interrater reliability, scaling properties, a linear regression and forecasting model, Rasch analysis, and concurrent validity on the LADS have been established and appear adequate. Formations in Health Care provides a LADS reference manual, training, credentialing of raters, a user's manual, a technical review of data submitted, and facility consultations. Data can be submitted via manual optical scan sheets, computer diskette, or interface with R/COM and Easter Seals systems. The cost of participation is $3,200, plus a sign on fee of $250/facility, $800 for training and credentialing, and $3/record for data processing. Discounts are available for larger providers and those using multiple Formations systems. Formations is aggregating approximately 22,000 records per year and had over 75,000 records in their acute rehabilitation database as of December 31, 1994. Most of the subscribers are free-standing rehabilitation hospitals, with HealthSouth being the major client. As of January 1, 1995, all subscribers have converted to using the FIM[SM] instead of the LADS, and some are also participating in UDS[MR][SM]. The main difference between the two systems is how the data are analyzed and presented. Formations uses the linear regression and forecasting model to show where the provider's results were in terms of the expected outcome (LOS and functional status) and provides sophisticated graphics that are helpful in marketing the rehabilitation programs. For more information contact Formations in Health Care at (312) 849-4200 or write to: Formations in Health Care, 155 N. Wacker Dr., Suite 725, Chicago, IL 60606.

PATIENT EVALUATION CONFERENCE SYSTEM (PECS)

The Patient Evaluation Conference System (PECS)[26,28,37,46] is operated by the Center for Rehabilitation Outcome Analysis and Marianjoy Rehabilitation Center in Weaton, IL. PECS contains over 140 defined and standardized items, and includes facility descriptors, patient demographics, referral source, referring physician, ICD-9 codes, functional diagnoses, level of care, program type, LOS, vocational status, and postdischarge needs. A user's manual, clinical instructional manual, software and software user manual, and technical and system support are provided to subscribers. The software program is designed on a relational database (dBase format) and provides users with interactive capabilities. Individual and summary reports, color graphic presentations, patient profiles, and narrative descriptions are provided. Customized analyses can be accomplished through an interface with SPSS, SAS, FoxPro, and other statistical programs. The average cost is $7,500 for the software license, $1,000 for training, and $1,150 for an annual licensing fee and technical support. There is an abundance of reliability and validity data on the PECS: interrater reliability, Rasch analysis, predictive validity/forecasting, measurement and scaling properties, and concurrent validity. Some of the PECS items provide the basis for functional status in the Ambulatory Patient Groups (APGs). The main difference between PECS and the preceding two systems (FIM[SM] and LADS) is that PECS was designed as a patient care conference planning and assessment tool. It provides an efficient means for reporting functional and medical status and progress at team conferences. Approximately 60 facilities are using the PECS system. Even though the software program is quite sophisticated, there is no comparative database or data management service offered to subscribers. For more information contact the Center on Outcome Analysis at Marianjoy Rehabilitation Hospital at (708) 462-4203.

REHABILITATION INSTITUTE OF CHICAGO–FUNCTIONAL ASSESSMENT SCALE VERSION 3 (RIC-FAS III)

RIC-FAS III[35] was implemented at the Rehabilitation Institute of Chicago on September 1, 1992. The inventory was designed to augment the FIM[SM] and provides over 80 items in the following disciplines/categories: Physical Medicine, Nursing, Occupational Therapy, Physical Therapy,

Psychology, Social Work, Communicative Disorders, Therapeutic Recreation, and Vocational Rehabilitation. The inventory includes measures of impairment, disability, and handicap. A Rasch analysis has established the measurement and scaling properties of the RIC-FAS III, and studies have shown good test–retest reliability and high correlations with the original FIM[SM] items. RIC-FAS '95 is under development and should be available by June 1995. For more information contact the Rehabilitation Institute of Chicago, 345 East Superior Street, Chicago, IL 60611; (312) 908-6000.

FUNCTIONAL ASSESSMENT MEASURE

The Functional Assessment Measure (FAM)[9] was developed by Santa Clara Valley Medical Center in 1988 and was designed specifically for brain injury, stroke, and neuro populations. The FAM consists of 12 items that have been added to the original 18 FIM items and are rated on the same 7-point scale. The FAM items include swallowing, car transfers, community mobility, reading, writing, speech intelligibility, emotional status, adjustment to limitations, employability, orientation, attention, and safety judgment. The FAM items emphasize the cognitive and psychosocial aspects of disability. When combined with the FIM[SM] items, the 30-item inventory provides a broader measure of level of disability and greater sensitivity for postacute rehabilitation functional assessment. Some of the FAM items also relate to community function. Interrater, interdisciplinary and interprocedural reliability of the FAM have been demonstrated. A Rasch analysis has been performed on the FAM, which demonstrated the interval and scaling properties of the FAM. The FAM also correlates with the FIM[SM], DRS, and other indices of severity. The inter-rater reliability of the attention and safety judgment items tended to be low. The FAM takes 25 to 35 minutes to complete and easily can be administered over the phone. The Traumatic Brain Injury (TBI) Model Projects, funded by the National Institute of Disability and Rehabilitation Research, have been using the FAM in combination with other clinical indicators. It is estimated there are over 200 rehabilitation facilities across the country who are using the FAM. Other than the TBI Model Project database, there is no means to compare outcomes between facilities. For more information contact the TBI project at Santa Clara Valley Medical Center at (408) 295-9896; 950 S. Bascom Avenue, Suite 2011, San Jose, CA 95128.

SUBACUTE REHABILITATION PROGRAMS

A subacute rehabilitation program can be located in an acute care hospital, a hospital-based skilled nursing facility, or a free-standing nursing facility. The patients served have expected outcomes of returning home or progressing to another level of rehabilitation care (e.g., comprehensive inpatient rehabilitation, outpatient, or home health).

HOSPITAL-BASED SUBACUTE PROGRAMS

According to CARF, three patients in Category II are generally cared for in acute care hospitals and have:

- variable risk of potential medical instability

- regular, direct individual contact with rehabilitation physicians determined by their medical and rehabilitation needs

- multiple and/or complex rehabilitation nursing needs and a potential for needing high medical acuity-skilled nursing

- a daily minimum of 1 to 3 hours of therapy from the interdisciplinary team

- education and training opportunities for themselves and their family on an ongoing basis.

SKILLED NURSING-BASED SUBACUTE PROGRAMS

Patients in category III

- have a lower risk of medical instability

- have less need for high medical acuity skilled nursing

- are usually treated in subacute rehabilitation programs.

These programs are usually operated in a skilled nursing facility (SNF), hospital-based or free-standing, that is certified as a Medicare Distinct Part SNF. JCAHO, in its 1995 *Survey Protocol for Subacute Programs,* defined *subacute care* as goal-oriented, comprehensive, inpatient care designed for an individual who has had an illness, injury, or exacerbation of a disease process. Subacute care is generally more intensive than traditional skilled nursing facility care and less intensive than acute care. Patients may be medically complex, with multiple medical conditions requiring close monitoring and treatment, or may have other conditions that may prevent them from tolerating the 3 hours of intensive therapy that are required in acute comprehensive inpatient rehabilitation. Additionally, many of the managed care companies are diverting acute rehabilitation patients to less intensive and less costly subacute rehabilitation programs.

DEFINING THE LEVEL OF CARE

Since many of the subacute facilities provide both medical and rehabilitation subacute programs, it is important to define the scope, intensity and capabilities of each level of care. There often are characteristic differences in the type and intensity of programs, nursing care hours, therapy, and services provided that can affect both costs and outcomes. There also appears to be differences between hospital-based and SNF-based subacute programs in terms of the caseload composition and medical acuity of patients. Generally, 60–80 percent of the subacute patients are rehabilitation (mostly stroke and orthopedic conditions), and 20–40 percent are medical cases (cardiac, pulmonary, wound, infectious diseases, complex medical, and postoperative conditions) whose primary program emphasis is skilled nursing and medical management. Subacute rehabilitation and subacute medical patients should be separated from an outcomes and quality management standpoint.

USING OUTCOME INDICATORS IN SUBACUTE PROGRAMS

The most commonly reported outcome indicators by subacute providers are average length of stay (ALOS) and percent discharged home. However, few providers break down this data by impairment group. Some subacute providers have been using modified versions of the FIM[SM] without established reliability and UDSMR[SM] credentialing of the FIM[SM] raters. Some of the larger nursing home chains such as Beverly, Hillhaven, NovaCare, Integrated Health, and GranCare have developed their own outcome systems, but they cannot compare results to other providers outside their system. Many of the subacute providers find that the Minimum Data Set (MDS)[236] and the 1987 OBRA requirements for SNFs are just not appropriate for the subacute rehabilitation patients whose ALOS is 19–20 days.

A number of organizations have set up databases that can be useful for subacute providers, including UDS$_{MR}$[SM], Formations in Health Care, Integrated Health Systems, Inc.,Beverly Enterprises, and Outcomes Management Services.

UDS$_{MR}$[SM] SUBACUTE DATA BASE

In 1992, UDS$_{MR}$[SM] established a separate data base for SNF/Rehabilitation subacute providers[242], using the FIM[SM] and other data elements in the UDS$_{MR}$[SM] system. Providers must be Medicare Distinct Part SNF rehabilitation providers, and/or a subacute program accredited by either JCAHO or CARF. There are currently over 100 subscribers to the UDS$_{MR}$[SM] subacute database, and 43 fully credentialed facilities are submitting data to UDS$_{MR}$[SM]. There are over 12,000 records in the UDS$_{MR}$[SM] subacute data base as of December 31, 1994. Subscribers are required to have a separate UDS$_{MR}$[SM] Facility Services Agreement, and the fees are the same as those for acute rehabilitation. UDS$_{MR}$[SM] offers subscribing facilities the UDS$_{MR}$[SM] Guide version 4.0, educational and training materials, questions and answers about the FIM[SM], regional and on-site FIM[SM] training and workshops, and the FIMware[TM] software program. To ensure reliable and accurate reporting of data, each facility goes through the same two-phase UDS$_{MR}$[SM] credentialing process as used with the acute rehabilitation providers.

Although the FIM[SM] and UDS$_{MR}$[SM] data set appear appropriate for subacute rehabilitation programs, the validity and reliability of the FIM[SM] for these programs are currently being evaluated. Aside from differences in caseload, medical acuity, FIM[SM] admit scores and FIM[SM] gains, it is important to monitor program interruptions, medical complications, transfers back to acute care, discharge destinations, and subsequent hospitalizations. For more information contact UDS$_{MR}$[SM] at (716) 829-2076 or write to: Uniform Data Systems for Medical Rehabilitation, 232 Parker Hall, State University of New York at Buffalo, 3435 Main St., Buffalo, NY 14214-3007.

FORMATIONS IN HEALTH CARE SUBACUTE REHABILITATION DATABASE

Similar to UDS$_{MR}$[SM], Formations in Health Care[231] established a separate database for subacute rehabilitation in 1993 using the same data elements and outcome indicators in the LADS system. In January 1995 they converted to using the FIM[SM] as the primary outcome indicator. There were 25 subscribers and 3,000 records submitted to the Formations subacute rehabilitation database as of December 31, 1994. Formations plans to develop a severity-adjusted forecast model using linear regression, similar to the one established for the acute rehabilitation database. Interrater reliability has been established, and raters have been credentialed and trained on the rating scales by Formations. Providers will be able to compare their results to the expected outcomes based on this model. Subscriber fees are the same as those established for the Formations' LADS system.

INTEGRATED HEALTH SYSTEMS, INC.

Integrated Health Systems has been using a combination of the FIM[SM] and the RIC-FAS II for their rehabilitation subacute and medically fragile populations. Since Integrated specializes in ventilatordependent and medically complex/fragile cases, their patients tend to be of higher medical acuity. Some of the outcome measures used may not be suitable for the subacute rehabilitation patient populations served by other facilities. However, Integrated has been collecting a wealth of outcome data for several years and has over 200,000 records in its database. They currently are focusing on better utilization of their own outcome data for program management and quality improvement, and developing global outcome indicators for their HIV programs. The major outcome indicators are used for all Integrated programs include:

- measures of wellness, general health perception (SF-36)
- rehospitalizations, program interruptions
- FIM^{SM}/RIC-FAS II
- discharge disposition (exclusive of hospice and medically unstable)
- nosocomial infections
- quality of life and global health status

REHABILITATION OUTCOME MEASURE (ROM)

Puls Point Technologies, a subsidiary of South Coast Rehabilitation Services (a contract therapy provider and subacute program management company), has developed an outcome indicator system called Rehabilitation Outcome Measure (ROM). The ROM is a discipline-specific outcome system that uses a 7-point rating scale, similar to the FIM^{SM}. It was developed by clinicians for functional deficits most commonly seen in subacute care.

In addition, Pulse Point Technologies has developed and licensed a fully integrated management information system for subacute and long-term-care programs called the OMS Network (which includes clinical documentation, outcome, quality, financial, marketing, and executive information). The outcome system currently is used in over 200 sites, including some Regency Health Services, Beverly Enterprises, Living Centers of America, Transitional Hospitals, and South Coast Rehabilitation Services facilities. Reliability and validity testing is in process, and a credentialing program has been established to maintain interrator reliability. For further information, contact Dan Larson at (800) 743-2810.

BEVERLY ENTERPRISES, INC.

Beverly Enterprises is using the Outcomes Management Services (OMS) network in many of its rehabilitation programs. Beverly's approach is to use global outcome measures, rather than individual measures designed for specific subacute populations. However, the reliability and validity of these measures have not been established.

SUBACUTE MEDICAL PROGRAMS

There are only a few outcome measures and systems available that might be appropriate for subacute medical programs. The majority of the caseload are medically complex, wound, cardiac, pulmonary, infectious diseases, metabolic disorders, or postoperative cases. Although the primary emphasis of subacute medical programs is on skilled nursing and medical management, some of these patients may receive up to an hour of therapy per day or every other day.

FORMATIONS IN HEALTH CARE MEDICAL OUTCOME SYSTEM

Formations in Health Care recently has developed a Medical Outcome System (MOS)[52,234] for chronic diseases, pain, wound, and respiratory treatment. Nine subacute provider systems participated in and funded this development: Arbor Health Care, Health Care Retirement, Hillhaven, Medbridge/Manor Health Care, Mediplex/Sunrise, Genesis Health Ventures, HealthSouth, Horizon, and Olympus Health Care Groups. Pilot testing of the instruments was completed in December 1994. An item analysis and Rasch analysis were performed, the inventories were condensed, and the scales were subsequently revised. Interrater reliability was established and appears adequate.

Demographics. The demographic data elements in the inventories are the same, and will default to the MDS or UDS$_{MR}^{SM}$ where there is overlap. A draft of the data collection forms has been developed. The demographics are shown below.

DEMOGRAPHICS OF THE FORMATIONS MEDICAL OUTCOME SYSTEM

Patient ID	Payment Source	Rehabilitation Impairment Group
Facility ID	Other Payment Source	Program Interruption
Corporate ID	Managed Care Product	Days of Program Interruptions
Admit Date	Managed Care Cost Control	Discharge Location
Zip Code	Strategy	Living With
Years of Education	Referral Source	Work Capability at Discharge
Ethnicity/Race	Pre-Admit Vocational Category	Total Billed Charges
Marital Status	Date Last Worked	Total Billed Therapy Charges
Birth Date	Admit From	Clinical Rating Forms Completed
Gender	Living With	Patient Follow-Up Contact
Major Surgical Procedures	Discharge Date	Method of Follow-Up
ICDM-9 Procedure Code	Primary ICDM-9 Code	Patient Phone Number
Date of Surgical Procedure	Date of Onset of Primary ICD-9	Second Phone Number/Contact
First Admission to Facility for Dx	Secondary ICDM-9 Code	
Number of Admissions	Date of Onset of Secondary ICD-9	
	Secondary ICD-9 codes (up to 5)	

Efficiency Measures. The efficiency measures include:

- LOS/visits

- charges/costs

- utilization of resources after discharge.

Effectiveness Measures. The effectiveness measures for the Formations MOS are shown below.

EFFECTIVENESS MEASURES FOR FORMATIONS MOS

Respiratory Treatment	**Wound Treatment**	**Pain Treatment**
Weaning dates	Total number of wounds	Worst pain
Resource utilization	Surface area by 5 criteria	Least pain
oxygen	Type of wound	Current pain
tracheostomy	Stages of wounds	Duration of pain
ventilator	Perimeter involvement	Pain interference with daily
Health status (dyspnea)		activities or quality of life
Oxygen saturation		measured by 5 criteria
Oxygen utilization		Pain treatment modalities
		and frequency

Outcome Measures. Ratings on the FIM[SM], IADL (instrumental activities of daily living), and Rancho Levels of Cognitive Function (LCFS)[12] are completed for all subacute rehabilitation patients. There is also a global health status and a measure of medical acuity status, which defines comorbidities and measures systemic disease for chronic disease patients on a 5-point scale, as follows:

- no systemic disease

- mild systemic disease

- systemic disease limits activity

- incapacitating disease

- moribund patient.

Formations currently is testing and revising the inventories, developing data collection forms and a certification training program. There currently are nine subscribers (subacute provider systems) to the MOS and 500 records in the database. A number of contracts with other subacute medical providers also are pending. The costs of participation are $2,400/ year for quarterly reports, plus a sign on fee of $250/facility, $1,000 for training and credentialing, and $3.50/record for data processing. Discounts are available for larger providers and those using multiple Formations systems. The MOS system is now available to other subacute providers through Formations in Health Care. There are about 75 subacute providers using the MOS program.

Formations plans to develop a severity-adjusted forecast model and to continue developing outcome measures for the other subacute medical populations. It is their hope to become the benchmark (goal standard) for subacute medical outcomes. For further information contact Formations in Health Care, 155 N. Wacker Drive, Suite 725, Chicago, IL 60606; (312) 849-4200.

SPINAL CORD INJURY PROGRAMS

There have been a diversity of outcome measures for spinal cord injury (SCI) programs proposed, everything from greater independence in ADL and mobility to better quality of life. The WHO[245] model and definitions of *impairment, disability, and handicap* provide a conceptual model for better understanding the various outcome measures and what they attempt to measure for spinal cord injury populations.

MEASURES OF IMPAIRMENT

The American Spinal Injury Association (ASIA)[218] developed measurement standards and guidelines in 1982 that focused primarily on measures of impairment. The ASIA Motor Score provides an assessment of highest and lowest motor and sensory function for each of 10 muscle groups by side of body. The ASIA Impairment (modified Frankel Class) Scale describes the degree of motor and sensory involvement upon admission (A–E). Both of these scales are examples of *impairment* measures.

MEASURES OF DISABILITY AND HANDICAP

Measures of *disability* in SCI have not been as well standardized as measures of impairment. Early efforts to measure disability focused on activities of daily living scales such as the Barthel Index.[33] The Quadriplegic Index of Function[224] is an expanded measure of ADL similar to the Barthel, but is designed to provide a more sensitive index of functional improvements in quadriplegics. Independence on 46 items is rated on a 5-point scale. In addition, a 20-item multiple-choice instrument tests for understanding of personal care needs. A similar scale, which was developed at Santa Clara Valley Medical Center in 1989, includes all of the FIM[SM] items and a parallel assessment of the ability to instruct others to carry out and perform the functions for the patient (if at an FIM[SM] level 3 or lower). The Rehabilitation Indicators Project[23] at NYU Medical Center provides measures of disability on hundreds of *skill indicators* (SKIs) for SCI, as well as *activity pattern indicators* (APIs) within the broader context of social roles. The Self-Observation and Report Technique (SORT)[221] is similar to the APIs and provides a measure of actual behaviors in the environment using a diary format. Both the APIs and SORT provide a sophisticated measure of *handicap* in SCI. The Craig Handicap Assessment Reporting Technique (CHART), described in detail later in this section, measures the level of handicap in the community.

REHABILITATION

The terms *medical rehabilitation* and *psychosocial rehabilitation* as defined by Alexander and Fuhrer[219] provide an additional framework to understanding the rehabilitation process and expected outcomes for SCI. Medical rehabilitation concentrates on the disablement phase from impairment to disability, with the goal of minimizing disability for a given degree of impairment. In SCI this means minimizing disabilities in personal care, locomotion, body disposition, and dexterity for a given level of lesion. Psychosocial rehabilitation concentrates on the disablement from disability to handicap with the goal of minimizing handicap for a given degree of disability. In SCI this means minimizing handicaps in physical function, role fulfillment, occupation, social integration, and economic self-sufficiency.

CRAIG HANDICAP ASSESSMENT REPORTING TECHNIQUE (CHART)

The Craig Handicap Assessment and Reporting Technique[223], developed by Whiteneck et al. in 1992, assesses physical independence, mobility, occupation, social integration, and economic self-sufficiency. The psychometric properties, reliability, and validity of the CHART have been demonstrated and are adequate. Designed as an interview or survey, CHART assesses the extent of handicap for individuals living in the community, regardless of number of years since injury or the extent of their involvement in the health care system. Rasch analysis of the CHART has demonstrated that it is a well-calibrated linear scale with good fit between the items.

NATIONAL SCI DATABASE

The National SCI Database was first established at the National Spinal Cord Injury Data Research Center for the 17 Model SCI systems funded by the National Institute of Disability and Rehabilitation Research (NIDRR) and was later transferred to the National Spinal Cord Injury Statistical Center (NSCISC) at the University of Alabama, Birmingham. The number of NIDR-funded Model SCI systems was reduced from 17 to 13 in 1985. These comprehensive care systems are designed to serve SCI persons from time of injury through acute and initial rehabilitation to a lifetime of follow-up care. There are currently over 16,000 records in the National SCI Database, with over 75,000 follow-up assessments as of December 31, 1994. The database includes measures of:

- impairment (ASIA Motor Scores, and standards for neurological classification)
- disability (FIM[SM])
- handicap (CHART)
- health (medical complications and days hospitalized)
- satisfaction (index of life satisfaction)
- costs (medical expenses, physicians, attendant care, equipment, and lost wages).

For more information, contact NSCISC at (205) 934-3330 or write to: NSCISC, University of Alabama, Spain Rehabilitation Center, 1717 6th Ave., S., Birmingham, AL 35233.

BRAIN INJURY PROGRAMS

There has been a lot of effort spent on the development of outcome measures and systems for brain injury programs. Most of the measures tend to focus more on the psychosocial, cognitive, behavioral, life skills development, employability, and community reintegration aspects of recovery. A number of outcome measures have been designed specifically for traumatic brain injury (TBI) programs.[8,11] Measures can be classified as indices of severity of impairment, disability scales, rehabilitation indices (LOS, charges, client satisfaction, and self-determination), handicap, and community activities.

GLASGOW COMA SCALE

One of the most commonly used and accepted impairment measures in TBI is the Glasgow Coma Scale (GCS).[10,15] It is a simple, internationally used standard for assessing depth and duration of coma. It is designed to measure three aspects of behavior:

- motor responsiveness

- verbal performance

- eye opening.

The GCS is most appropriately applied within the first 24 hours following injury and can be used as a measure of severity of impairment. A GCS of 3–8 has been defined as a severe injury, 9–12 as moderate, and 13–15 as mild brain injury. There is an abundance of reliability and validity data available on GCS. Some investigators have attempted to improve on the GCS by adding items such as the Glasgow-Lege Scale, Coma Near-Coma Scale, Coma Recovery Scale, and Western Neuro-Sensory Stimulation Profile. Other indicators of severity may include the length of coma, duration of posttraumatic amnesia, and the Galveston Orientation and Amnesia Test (GOAT).

DISABILITY RATING SCALE (DRS)

The Disability Rating Scale (DRS)[9,14] was developed by Rappaport et al. in 1973 to measure general functional status and disability level from coma to community. The DRS consists of several items divided into four categories:

1. arousability, awareness, responsivity

2. cognitive ability for self-care activities

3. ability to depend on others

4. psychosocial adaptability.

The subitems include:

- eye opening

- communication ability

- motor response

- cognitive ability for self-care (feeding, toileting, grooming)

- overall level of function

- employability.

Interrater, interprocedural and interinformant reliability were high. Concurrent validity of the DRS has been well established, as well as predictive validity in terms of discharge disposition, return to work, and acute hospital length of stay. The DRS has been found to be a strong predictor of need for supervision and return to work 1 year postinjury. The DRS has also been applied to cerebrovascular accident (CVA) patients with some success. The advantage of the DRS is its relative ease of use both in terms of complexity and time required to complete the inventory (fewer than 10 minutes). The DRS has been shown to be an effective tool to track progress across the continuum of clinical services and the course of functional recovery. The drawbacks of the DRS include its assessment of general functioning rather than specific behavior, limited application in patients with only physical disability, and its sensitivity to extreme and mild TBI cases. The DRS has been used in multiple outcome studies and is part of the TBI Model Projects Data Base.

RANCHO LEVELS OF COGNITIVE FUNCTION SCALE (LCFS)

The Levels of Cognitive Function Scale (LCFS)[12] was developed at Rancho Los Amigos Hospital in 1972 and describes eight stages of cognitive function and recovery following a TBI. The eight cognitive levels on the Rancho Scale describe various levels of:

- responsiveness to stimuli and the environment

- responses to verbal commands

- alertness

- agitation

- purposeful and nonpurposeful behavior

- memory

- attention span

- verbalization

- functional independence

- insight

- judgment

- reasoning

- carry-over for new learning

- social behavior in a global description.

These are dimensions of behavior/function that are described in detail at each of the eight levels of cognitive function.

The LCFS has received international acceptance and is used as a screening tool and admission criteria for various programs and levels of care. The LCFS also is included in the TBI Model Systems Database.

FUNCTIONAL ASSESSMENT MEASURE (FAM)

The Functional Assessment Measure (FAM)[9], which was specifically designed for brain injury, stroke, and neuro populations, was described in a previous section on outcome measures for comprehensive inpatient rehabilitation programs. The TBI Model Projects funded by NIDRR have been using the FAM in combination with the DRS, GCS, LCFS and other clinical indicators for TBI.

COMMUNITY INTEGRATION QUESTIONNAIRE (CIQ)

The Community Integration Questionnaire (CIQ)[16] was developed as a measure of reduced handicap with TBI in the community. The CIQ contains 15 items, including participation in:

- household activities
- shopping
- errands
- leisure activities
- visiting friends
- social events
- productive activities.

The CIQ appears to be a viable measure of community integration for the TBI Model Systems and research on outcomes after TBI. It has adequate test–retest reliability, and high correlations between ratings of TBI individuals by therapy practitioners and by family members. Factor analysis has identified three related but distinct dimensions:

- home integration
- social integration
- productive activities.

The CIQ correlates significantly with the CHART, another handicap measure discussed previously. The CIQ takes approximately 10–15 minutes to complete and has been applied to TBI patients up to 6–7 years postinjury. The CIQ does not assess integration skills or deficits in skills. It also does not provide a fair assessment for patients who did not engage in the activities prior to injury. Despite its limitations, the CIQ currently is the best single and simple measure of community integration and handicap for TBI.

EMPLOYMENT AND PRODUCTIVE ACTIVITIES

Employment and productive activities are critical determinants of successful reintegration of a TBI individual into society. Employment or productive activities are important handicap measures and relatively easy to document. The FAM, DRS, and CIQ all contain some measure of employability. The RIC-FAS III also contains measures of community recreation integration, initiation and participation, leisure skills and awareness of community resources.

LIVING ARRANGEMENTS (DISPOSITION)

Living arrangements, and with whom, are factors strongly correlated with level of severity of disability and the need for supervision. They also provide some measure of the economic costs associated with TBI. The UDSmr[SM] system provides a coding schema for determining patients' living setting and who they are living with on admission, discharge, and follow-up from inpatient rehabilitation. The TBI Model Systems provide a more comprehensive listing of options. Hours of supervision or assisted care per day also can provide a measure of level of independence and functioning in the community.

LIFE SATISFACTION

Overall life satisfaction can be used as a global indicator of the impact of rehabilitation efforts with TBI individuals. Examples of life satisfaction measures include: Life Satisfaction Index-A[13], Quality of Life Scale[7], and Personal Well-Being Scale[8], none of which was developed specifically for TBI. Life satisfaction is known to be correlated with mood and may be affected by income level, adjustment to limitations and community living, recovery, and degree of perceived control over one's environment.

TBI MODEL SYSTEMS NATIONAL DATABASE

The TBI Model Systems funded by NIDRR established a national database for TBI patients in 1989. The five centers were reduced to four in 1991. The six criteria for subject inclusion are:

- individual has TBI with or without skull fracture as evidenced by:
  loss of consciousness, posttraumatic amnesia (PTA),
  objective neurological findings

- individual was admitted to the TBI Model System ER within 8 hours of injury

- individual was age 16 years or older at time of injury

- individual resides in designated catchment area of model system

- individual has acute care and rehabilitation within the system hospitals

- individual signs or family member or conservator signs informed consent to participate in study.

The national TBI data set includes over 300 items in the following categories:

- dates

- demographic data

- physical status descriptors (e.g., cause of injury, CT scan results, GCS, trauma score etc.)

- functional status descriptors (e.g., Neuropsych battery, DRS, FAM[SM], FIM, and LCFS)

- therapeutic interventions

- emergency medical services data

- follow-up assessment

- community integration (e.g., CIQ and other indicators).

Subjects are followed at the first 6 months and annually after discharge from inpatient rehabilitation up to 7 years postinjury. There are over 600 subjects in the TBI Model Systems national database, with over 900 follow-up assessments as of December 31, 1994. For more information, contact the Rehabilitation Institute of Michigan. ▪

9. OUTCOME MEASURES AND SYSTEMS FOR OUTPATIENT AND COMMUNITY-BASED SETTINGS

OUTPATIENT MEDICAL REHABILITATION PROGRAMS

There is a dearth of outcome measures specifically developed for outpatient rehabilitation programs. No one single measure will satisfy all of the outcome objectives and customer expectations for outpatient rehabilitation, which tends to include a relatively diverse population of clients with different impairments. Historically this is an area that has been neglected in outcome evaluation systems. However, there have been a number of recent developments in outcome measures for outpatient rehabilitation. The major focus of most outpatient services is on reducing *handicap*.

RESTORE—FORMATIONS IN HEALTH CARE (NEUROLOGIC OUTCOMES SYSTEM)

RESTORE[167], developed by Formations in Health Care, is an outcome evaluation system designed for comprehensive outpatient rehabilitation programs for neurological conditions (i.e., stroke, brain injury, spinal cord injury, and other neurological problems). RESTORE, which was released in August of 1992, contains the following:

- a condensed version of the SF–36 (a handicap health-related perception of wellness measure discussed later in this section)[95]

- demographic information (e.g., primary insurance, admitting and discharge residential status, age, gender, and comorbidities)

- units of service (e.g., physical therapy, occupational therapy, speech therapy, psychological therapy, or vocational therapy)

- ADL (e.g., dressing, grooming, toileting, washing/bathing, and feeding)

- community reentry skills (i.e., IADL and social involvement)

- communication skills (i.e., comprehension and expression)

- cognitive retraining (e.g., calculation, memory, problem solving, and self monitoring).

Functional status is rated on a 5-point scale, similar to the one used with the LADS scales. The 5-point scale appears more restrictive than the FIM[SM] 7-point scale, and it may not be sensitive enough to measure small increments of change in outpatient rehabilitation programs. Interrater reliability and the scaling properties of the RESTORE have been established. Validity studies are pending. There were 45 subscribers to Formation's RESTORE system contributing approximately 3,500 records annually as of December 31, 1994. The cost of participation is

$2,000/year for quarterly reports, plus a sign on fee of $250/facility, $1,500 for training and credentialing, and $3/record for data processing. Discounts are available for larger providers, and those using multiple Formations systems. RESTORE was renamed Neurologic Outcomes System in January 1995. Formations also is developing outcome systems for orthopedic and occupational outpatient rehabilitation programs. For more information call (312) 849-4200.

ORTHOPEDIC OUTCOME SCALE-FORMATIONS IN HEALTH CARE

Formations in Health Care has recently developed and released a draft of the proposed Orthopedic Outcome Scale[166], which has been field tested in six facilities. The inventory includes a modified version of the SF–36, patient satisfaction, strength, endurance, active ROM, functional goals, activity profile, pain, program completion, and services provided. Interrater reliability is being evaluated during the field test. The Orthopedic Outcome Scale is now available through Formations in Health Care. The price schedule is expected to be similar to RESTORE.

FOCUS ON THERAPEUTIC OUTCOMES, INC. (FOTO)

A consortium of outpatient rehabilitation providers including representatives from CareMark, Continental Medical Systems, HealthSouth, Med Rehabilitation, NovaCare—Outpatient Division, Rehabilitation, and Rehabilitation Clinics, Inc. formed FOTO[160] in 1993 to develop an outcome system for outpatient rehabilitation. FOTO's initial objectives were to

- develop a national standard to measure functional outcomes resulting from outpatient therapeutic interventions

- develop a means to measure the efficacy of therapy services

- establish of a provider database

- guide research and development of health care reform.

The outcome measures initially selected included the Evaluation of Knee Ligament Injuries[168], Neck Disability Index[169], Owestry Low Back Disability Evaluation[159] and the SF–36.[95] After a pilot phase of testing the various instruments, a factor analysis was done that revealed similar patterns and results on the three instruments. So all but a modified version of the SF–36 were dropped. The present FOTO inventory contains 30 items with a modified version of the SF–36 in the categories of role parameters, pain, physical functioning, and patient satisfaction. The mental health and depression components of the SF–36 also were dropped. The demographic data elements collected include:

- date of initial visit

- age

- sex

- gender

- ethnicity

- weight

- height

- Social Security Number

- primary ICD-9 and secondary ICD-9 codes

- date of onset

- surgical history

- referral source information.

Assessments of function are completed by both the patient and the clinician. No follow-up data are collected postdischarge.

The target populations for FOTO are back, neck, knee, arthritis, pain, and orthopedic patients. FOTO includes assessments by either a PT or an OT. Data are recorded and transmitted via optical scan sheets to the FOTO Data Management Service in Knoxville, TN. There currently are four major outpatient rehabilitation systems, representing 120 outpatient clinics and hospitals participating in FOTO. The costs of participation are $4,500/year for quarterly reports, plus a $5,000 initiation fee/company, $3,900 for optical scanner and software, and $3.75/record for electronic or $5.00/record for optical scan sheet data submission and processing. There are no built in quality controls for errors and omissions, accuracy of data submitted, or reliability or validity results on the FOTO system. For more information call (800) 482-FOTO or write to: FOTO, Inc., PO Box 11444, Knoxville, TN 37939.

SHORT FORM 36 (SF-36) AND THE MEDICAL OUTCOMES STUDY

Health status, quality of life, and the patient's perception of wellness measures have gained widespread acceptance among researchers as good measures to predict ongoing and future health care utilization for cardiac, pulmonary, HIV positive, back and neck pain, arthritis, and other medical conditions. The Short Form 36 (SF–36)[90,91,95,102] initially was developed out of the RAND corporation and the Medical Outcomes Study[82,83] as a measure of "patient perception of wellness." It taps eight health concepts:

- physical functioning

- bodily pain

- role limitations due to physical health problems

- role limitations due to personal or emotional problems

- emotional wellbeing

- social functioning

- energy/fatigue

- general health perceptions.

Although the SF–36 and subsequent versions have gained widespread acceptance as good measures to predict future health care utilization, they are not well suited for the disabled, particularly the geriatric disabled. Throughout their rehabilitation efforts, occupational therapy professionals try to teach patients and their families about the disabling condition(s), early signs of deterioration, and secondary medical complications. The SF–36 assesses whether there is a preoccupation with health-related concerns. Most disabled patients have a rather negative reaction to the SF–36, with feelings of despondency, depression, or lack of compliance in completing the forms. They tend to feel frustration and humiliation over the types of questions asked and the fear of being perceived as overly obsessed with health concerns. The occupational therapist may have taught the patients the proper body mechanics and posture to safely carry out an activity and what some of the signs or symptoms of improper body mechanics may be. Therefore, disabled patients are taught to pay more attention to their bodily functions, pain, and level of activity.

This negative reaction by disabled patients to the SF–36 certainly has been the experience of Formations in Health Care and other researchers who have attempted to incorporate a modified version of the SF–36 into their outcome measurement systems. A more appropriate measure for the disabled population might be satisfaction with life or satisfaction with adjustment (i.e., community adjustment, home living, progress and recovery, learning new ways of doing things, compensating for and coping with disability and handicap, and accepting their limitations). For more information on the SF–36, contact the Medical Outcomes Trust at (617) 426-4046 or write to Medical Outcomes Trust, 20 Park Plaza, Suite 1014, Boston, MA 02116-4313.

FUNCTIONAL ASSESSMENT SCREENING QUESTIONNAIRE (FASQ)

The Functional Assessment Screening Questions (FASQ)[163] was developed by Granger et al. in 1993 as an outcome measure for the combined outpatient rehabilitation medicine and family medicine primary care settings. The FASQ now is being field tested for other outpatient practice settings and home health settings. The FASQ was designed for the following target impairments:

- neuromusculoskeletal (upper limbs and neck, manual dexterity, lower limbs, and trunk)
- communication (speaking and writing)
- sensory (seeing, reading, and hearing)
- cardiopulmonary (stamina)
- cognitive
- affective.

The items cover personal activities of daily living, IADL, leisure, occupation, and transportation, plus four questions concerning general health and functioning. Reliability of self-report patient and family assessments appears adequate. A Rasch analysis, however, did not provide sufficient evidence that patients were being measured on the most appropriate scale. The FASQ shows promise, but further research is required.

PHYSICAL PERFORMANCE AND MOBILITY EXAM (PPME)

The Physical Performance and Mobility Exam (PPME)[165] was developed to measure functional mobility of the frail elderly while hospitalized and in the home setting during follow-up. The

PPME has been factored down to 6 principal items and can now be completed in less than 10 minutes. These items are:

- bed mobility

- transfers bed/chair

- strength/endurance/coordination

- balance

- balance/strength

- ambulation.

Items are scored on a pass/fail basis according to speed and efficiency and level of assistance required. Test–retest reliability was good, and interrater reliability was fair. The PPME was validated against other clinical indicators, but without conclusive results. The PPME may have limited application as an outcome measure in outpatient rehabilitation.

AMBULATORY PATIENT CLASSIFICATION SYSTEM (APG)

HCFA has contracted with the 3M Health Information System to develop an Ambulatory Patient Classification System (APGs)[157] designed to explain the amount and type of resources used in ambulatory care. APGs was developed to encompass the full range of ambulatory settings, including surgery units, hospitals and emergency departments, outpatient clinics, day hospitals, and home health. A total of 289 APGs have been identified based on the Major Diagnostic Categories (MDCs) from the DRG classification system, CPT codes, Relative Value Units (RVUs), and Signs, Symptoms, and Findings (SSFs). A series of V-codes (diagnostic and impairment codes), H-codes (health status and functioning), and SSFs were developed to refine the coding for ambulatory care. The Functional Health Status section, a component of the H-codes, is intended for use in reporting the functional status of rehabilitation patients, mental patients, and patients with chronic diseases. There are 50 items in this section, which is based on a modification of the PECS system. Items are grouped into Self-Care, Sphincter Control, Locomotion, Cognition and Social Integration, Community Integration, Pain, Communication, and Adaptive Equipment. A 4-point rating scale is used for the Sphincter Control, Cognition, Community Integration, and Pain items; a 5-point scale is used for the Self-Care, Locomotion, and Mobility items; and a 7-point scale is used for the Communication items. Reliability, validity, and scaling properties of this modified inventory have not been demonstrated for outpatient rehabilitation programs. The New York Sate Department of Health currently is field testing the instruments and validating the APG model. Given the nature of the APG project, and the involvement of 3M and HCFA in developing this system for ambulatory care, serious consideration should be given to the potential use of this outcome measure for geriatric and orthopedic rehabilitation outpatients. [Health Information Systems, 3M Health Care, 100 Barnes Road, PO Box 5007, Wallingford, CT 06492-7507; 203-949-0303.]

OCCUPATIONAL REHABILITATION PROGRAMS

CARF defines occupational rehabilitation programs as comprehensive, outcome-oriented programs designed to minimize risk and optimize work capabilities of persons served. Work-specific occupational rehabilitation programs incorporate real or simulated work tasks into the individualized treatment program. The minimum required for program evaluation systems are specified in Chapter 4.

Work and productive activities represent a major category of performance areas for occupational therapy practitioners. Work-hardening programs differ in size, staff, equipment, program emphasis (types of work simulation), method, and services. An individual's motivation to return to work may depend on policies regarding worker's compensation, disability benefits, pending litigation, additional sources of income, local market and labor conditions, and many other socioeconomic factors. It is difficult to make fair comparisons of outcomes among programs. As with most outpatient rehabilitation programs, the main focus is on handicap issues, capacity, and productivity. There have been only a few outcome measures designed specifically for occupational rehabilitation or work-hardening programs.

OCCUPATIONAL OUTCOME SCALE-FORMATIONS IN HEALTH CARE

Formations in Health Care has recently developed the Occupational Outcome Scale[82] and has field tested the instrument in 25 occupational rehabilitation and work-hardening programs. Interrater reliability, validity, and psychometric properties have been established and appear adequate. The Occupational Outcome Scale is now available through Formations in Health Care. The inventory contains an assessment of physical demands and capacity in

- standing

- walking

- sitting

- lifting

- carrying

- pushing/pulling

- climbing

- stooping/crouching/kneeling

- reaching

- handling/fingering.

These items are rated on a 4-point scale by both the patient and the clinician on admission. The inventory also contains

- a modified version of the SF-36 (completed by the patient)

- an assessment of behavior demands and potential for return to work (assessed by the clinician)

- Follow-up information about employment, vocational status, earnings, and productive activities (collected from the patient at 90 days after program completion).

The price schedule is expected to be similar to RESTORE. For more information call (312) 849-4200 or write to: Formations in Health Care, 155 North Wacker Dr., Suite 725, Chicago, IL 60606.

WORK AND INDUSTRIAL REHABILITATION EVALUATION (WIRE)

The Work and Industrial Rehabilitation Evaluation (WIRE)[80,83] is an outcome evaluation system developed at 22 work-hardening programs in the Wisconsin Work Programs Network over a 2-year period from 1991 to 1992. Data were gathered and analyzed on 928 clients discharged from these programs, who had mostly lumbar and cervical spine injuries and carpal tunnel syndrome. Length of treatment was measured in weeks and number of visits. Client outcomes were based on return to work criteria in 10 different categories. Comparisons were made between length of treatment and client outcome for the major conditions treated. Based on this initial study, the WIRE system was developed. It collects data in 19 different categories as shown below.

CATEGORIES FOR THE WIRE SYSTEM

Gender

Age

Occupational category

Payment sources

Referral source

Diagnosis/injury site

Activities (i.e., functional assessment, situational assessment, physical capacity, job analysis, education and prevention, work modification, stress management, vocational assessment, symptom control, work hardening, work conditioning, occupational therapy, and physical therapy)

Time from onset of injury

Last day of work

Time from discharge to return to work

Number of program days

Duration of treatment/day

Length of treatment (weeks)

Psychological service

Surgery performed

Vocational services

Medical management

Patient outcomes (i.e., return to job, workload/job modifications, alternative job, alternative job with modifications, change in occupation, referred to vocational services, retired, medical referral, school, laid off, or other)

Total costs of treatment

WIRE provides an IBM-based software program to collect and analyze the data on the 19 variables and produce quarterly and annual reports. The cost of the software program is $150 for AOTA members and $250 for non-AOTA members. There is no data management service or comparative database established at this time. For more information, contact AOTA Products at (800) SAY-AOTA or write to: AOTA Products, 4720 Montgomery Lane, PO Box 31220, Bethesda, MD 20824-1220.

EARLY INTERVENTION AND PRESCHOOL DEVELOPMENT PROGRAMS

Early intervention and preschool development programs are structured to facilitate early child development through prevention, education, and therapeutic services for children with disabilities or who are at risk of developmental delays and to provide supportive educational/therapeutic services for their families. This includes infants and children with congenital deformities (e.g., spina bifida, Down's syndrome, cerebral palsy), developmental disabilities, and learning disabilities and children who are at risk of developmental delays due to abnormal birth circumstances, weight, or metabolic and neurological function. Performance components of occupational therapy interventions may focus on sensory-motor simulation, motor-perceptual skills, postural control, adaptive and assistive devices, seating, neuromuscular facilitation, parent skills in play and motivation, and modification of play activities. The ultimate goal of such programs in early childhood and educational development is to minimize any delays or the effects of disabilities and handicaps. Outcomes, therefore, can be divided into

- infant or early child outcomes
- parent outcomes
- parent–child and family outcomes
- educational outcomes
- costs
- community impact.[57]

The Accreditation Council[1] has switched to client-based outcome standards and offers some additional guidelines on the selection and development of appropriate client outcome measures for children with disabilities.

CHILD OUTCOMES

Most of the existing developmental scales have been standardized on normal children and are not easily normed for children with congenital deformities or development disabilities.[57] Instead of a norm-referenced approach, the choice may be to use a criteria-referenced test that evaluates the child's performance with respect to defined and expected behaviors that are appropriate for that child's age, impairment, and level of disability. Most infant tests rely heavily on motor behaviors that can discriminate among infants with motor dysfunction. The presence of abnormal muscle tone or reflexes can obscure test results. IQ or DQ scores, although clinically useful, provide poor outcome measures of a child's performance. Outcome measures that focus on socioemotional development, medical management, behavior management, independence, and physical growth have received recent attention.

WEEFIM[SM]

The Functional Independence Measure for Children (WeeFIM[SM])[67], which is part of UDS$_{MR}$[SM], was designed for children from 6 months to 7 years of age. The WeeFIM[SM] includes the same 18 FIM[SM] items, rated on a 7-point scale that takes into account the growth and developmental stages. Motor subscale, cognitive subscale and total WeeFIM[SM] norms are included in the WeeFIM[SM] Guide, which was released by UDS$_{MR}$[SM] in 1994. The initial reliability and validity data from the pilot test of the WeeFIM[SM] with 200 children demonstrated promising results. A Rasch analysis further demonstrated the scaling properties, fit of items, weighting, and discriminative ability among children with different impairments. The WeeFIM[SM] also correlated significantly with scores on the Battelle Development Screening Inventory Test[63] and the Vineland Adaptive Behavior Scales.[65] There currently are over 80 subscribers, including pediatric programs enrolled in CHAMPUS, who are using the WeeFIM[SM]. For more information on the WeeFIM[SM], contact Susan Braun at (716) 829-2076 or write to Braun at Uniform Data System for Medical Rehabilitation, State University of New York at Buffalo, 232 Parker Hall, 3435 Main St., Buffalo, NY 14214-3007.

PARENT OUTCOMES

A parent's psychological status and adjustment can be an important measure of outcomes. Measures of parenting stress and resources also have proven helpful.[62] Parents' reaction to a disabled child and their attribution of cause or responsibility can set the stage for how they interact and develop together.

PARENT–CHILD AND FAMILY OUTCOMES

A parent's view of his or her child is based on a comparison of the child's behavior against the parent's expectations. These expectations can strongly affect a child's subsequent development. Parent–child interactions and parenting techniques can be important motivators or deterrents for a child's behavior. Recently, there have been some encouraging attempts to apply family systems theories to the study of families with severely disabled children.[66]

EDUCATIONAL OUTCOMES

A school-aged child with a congenital deformity or developmental or learning disability receives an Individualized Education Plan (IEP) that is customized to his or her unique needs. An IEP includes:

- clinical assessments
- family goals and expectations
- therapeutic intervention and services required
- special educational programs and modifications
- adaptive physical education.

The educational objectives established in the IEP can be used as a proxy for educational outcomes.

COSTS AND COMMUNITY IMPACT

The costs and community impact of disabled children who do not receive appropriate and effective early intervention and preschool development can be considerable. One approach to measuring the cost-effectiveness of these programs includes an assessment of the cost savings of remedial education, extended therapy intervention, social services, and correctional services. Keeping these disabled children out of institutions can be another measure of community impact.

COMMUNITY REENTRY PROGRAMS

Community reentry or community living programs are residential facilities with structured programs designed to develop the necessary cognitive, behavioral, social, and life skills to enable clients to be successfully reintegrated into the community. The programs may be integrated into a client's home or community. Integrated living programs such as supervised living, supported independent living, or family living programs are offered in homes in which the client chooses to live. Congregate living programs provide residential services in larger facilities that are generally self-contained and can accommodate 8 to 16 clients. CARF, in its 1995 Standards Manual, now refers to both of these as community support services, which is a broader concept incorporating:

- personal, social, and community supports

- family supports

- host family supports

- respite supports

- living supports.

Community reentry or community living programs are designed to facilitate the transition of people with severe disabilities from a structured and comparatively dependent living situation to one in which they are more independent in the community.[19] The primary services provided include skill training in

- attendant care

- financial management

- consumer affairs

- mobility

- educational and vocational opportunities

- medical needs

- living arrangements

- social skills

- time management

- functional life skills

- sexuality.

With increased emphasis being placed on personal rights and self-determination, these community reentry and community living programs have begun to pay more close attention to the client's role in decision making and to client-centered outcomes.

Researchers have used a wide variety of techniques for assessing an individual's level of independence, including

- psychological measures

- functional measures

- social and behavioral measures

- multiple measures and inventories.

The more commonly used outcome measures for community reentry or community living programs are described here.

PSYCHOLOGICAL MEASURES

The California Psychological Inventory and the 16 Personality Factors Questionnaire (16 PF)[251] have been used in studies of independence.[20,21] The 16 PF provides a measure of "subduedness vs. independence" that is derived from a formula using 10 scores on selected factors of the inventory. Reliability and predictive validity of the 16 PF have been demonstrated for this population. [Available through Western Psychological Services, 12031 Wilshire Blvd., Los Angeles, CA 90025-1251; 800-648-8857.]

FUNCTIONAL MEASURES

The Barthel Index and FIM[SM], described earlier, appear to have relevance and application to community living programs. The Functional Assessment Inventory (FAI)[247] is a 39-item inventory that includes global measures of independence in the areas of

- learning ability

- sensory functioning

- physical functioning

- health status

- economic situation

- judgment

- problem solving

- initiative

- personality characteristics.

SOCIAL AND BEHAVIORAL MEASURES

Independence as a social factor has been operationally defined in the independent living (IL) movement and programs.[22] It includes such variables as

- mobility at home or in the community

- use of public transportation

- ADL

- use of personal care attendants

- adaptive equipment

- communication abilities

- source and amount of income

- living arrangement

- employment status

- educational level

- use of leisure time

- health status

- marital status

- social life

- self-concept.

Many of the variables have both functional and social cognitive components that can be isolated. The definition of independence focuses on the psychological and social factors. The IL inventory has been relatively widely used in independent living centers, regardless of setting or program type. Reliability of IL has been adequate, and the predictive validity in terms of successful reintegration into community and productive activities has been demonstrated. The IL was developed by Lachat and Williams (1984) and information is available from the Center for Resource Management, East Kingston, NH.

VOCATIONAL REHABILITATION PROGRAMS

Vocational rehabilitation (VR) programs provide a comprehensive process that systematically uses work (real or simulated) as the focal point for assessment and vocational exploration and counseling, with the ultimate goal of vocational adjustment and reemployment. Vocational evaluation incorporates medical, psychological, social, vocational, cultural, and economic factors (performance contexts) into the planning of vocational goals, objectives and recommended services, and training. CARF includes vocational evaluation under the broader category of employment services, which also includes community employment services, job placement, occupational skill training, work adjustment, and/or work services. Occupational skill training is often an integral part of a vocational rehabilitation program. The minimum criteria for a program evaluation system for community employment services are identified in Section IV. However, these criteria apply to only to employment and employment-related programs and services. The most commonly used outcome measures in vocational rehabilitation programs are described below.

FUNCTIONAL ASSESSMENT INVENTORY (FAI)

The Functional Assessment Inventory (FAI)[247], described briefly under community reentry and living programs, originally was designed to assess VR clients' potential for reemployment. It consists of 30 items measuring functional limitations and 10 items assessing strength and endurance. The descriptions of each item and scale emphasize vocationally pertinent skills and behaviors. In addition to the functional limitations (FL) score, the FAI can be scored on seven factors:

- adaptive behavior

- motor functioning

- cognition

- physical condition

- communication

- vocational qualifications

- vision.

Interrater reliability, interinformant reliability, and predictive validity in terms of future work status and earnings have been clearly demonstrated. The FAI also has been translated into a self-report inventory for clients.

HUMAN SERVICE SCALE (HSS)

The Human Service Scale (HSS)[249] was designed to assess a client's rehabilitation needs as a basis for providing appropriate rehabilitation services and determining whether the services were effective. The 80-item inventory requires either biographical information or self-report from clients and is scored on seven factors that closely resemble Maslow's hierarchy of needs. The validity of HSS with VR clients has been demonstrated, and there were high correlations with components of the MMPI (Minnesota Multiphasic Personality Inventory).

MINNESOTA SATISFACTION QUESTIONNAIRE (MSQ)

The Minnesota Satisfaction Questionnaire (MSQ)[253] was designed to measure a client's satisfaction with 20 different aspects of the work environment including:

- ability utilization

- achievement

- advancement

- coworkers

- independence and autonomy

- variety

- work conditions.

The 100-item inventory has been condensed through factor analysis to 20 items. Internal consistency of the 20 items was high, and test–retest reliability and concurrent validity were good.[253]

MINNESOTA SATISFACTORINESS SCALES (MSS)

The MSS[248] is similar to the MSQ and provides a measure of the employer's satisfaction with the client's job performance. The 28-item multiple choice inventory can be completed by the employee's supervisor in about 5 minutes. Score are calculated on four subscales:

- performance

- conformance

- personal adjustment

- dependability.

Internal consistency of the items appears high, but test–retest reliability adjusting for changes in performance level was poor. The MSS clearly discriminates between satisfactory and unsatisfactory workers who are likely to leave their jobs.

MINNESOTA SURVEY OF EMPLOYMENT EXPERIENCES (MSEE)

The MSEE[252] is a follow-up self-report measure designed to be completed by the VR client without professional assistance. The MSEE collects information about

- work experience prior to VR services

- work experience from case closure to follow-up contact

- details about current employment situation

- related vocational information such as the influence of handicap on job search success.

There are no reliability data available on the MSEE other than its perceived usefulness.

SERVICE OUTCOME MEASUREMENT FORM (SOMF)

SOMF[254] is a counselor rating instrument designed for state or federal VR counselors. Six domains or areas of function of VR clients are assessed:

- difficulty

- education

- economic–vocational status

- physical functioning

- adjustment to disability

- social competency.

The SOMF can be completed in fewer than 10 minutes. Interrater reliability of the items is adequate, and predictive validity appears good.

SIXTEEN PERSONALITY FACTOR QUESTIONNAIRE FORM E (16 PF-E)

The 16 PF[251] was described briefly under community reentry and living programs and is a self-report personality inventory designed for persons with limited educational or cultural backgrounds. It also has been used for a variety of rehabilitation populations, including mentally retarded adults, clients with schizophrenia, and VR clients. The 16 PF measures 16 primary dimensions of normal personality function, including warmth, dominance, sensitivity, imagination, insecurity, self-sufficiency, extroversion, adjustment, toughmindedness, independence, and discipline. Parallel form reliability and internal consistency of items were good.

WORK PERSONALITY PROFILE (WPP)

The WPP[250] is an observer rating instrument of situational assessments and job performance of VR clients. It consists of 58 items, each of which is rated on a 4-point scale of work performance. The 11 work performance subscales include: acceptance of work, ability to profit from instruction, work role, work tolerance, amount of supervision required, training assistance, anxiety/comfort with supervisor, relationship with supervisor, ability to socialize with coworkers, and communications skills. Internal consistency of items in the inventory and within subscales was high, and interrater agreement was low.

PSYCHIATRIC REHABILITATION PROGRAMS

Psychiatric rehabilitation programs and chemical dependency programs have grown in popularity and scope over the last 2 decades. Psychiatric rehabilitation programs are organized to develop, support, and maximize the quality of life and functional abilities of persons with severe and/or persistent psychiatric disorders, with the ultimate goal of successfully reintegrating them back into society.

Psychiatric rehabilitation programs may be categorized into

- inpatient psychiatric programs

- partial hospitalization programs

- residential treatment programs

- community housing programs

- outpatient therapy services

- emergency or crisis intervention services.

(Note that psychiatric programs can be inpatient or outpatient, and thus also could have been included in Chapter 8.)

CARF has developed requirements for a program evaluation system for all of the preceding program types in its 1995 *Standards for Mental health Programs*. See the following pages for these program evaluation standards.

The American Association of Partial Hospitalization (AAPH)[194] has developed an outcome measurement protocol for ambulatory mental health services that defines an essential set of variables to be measured; identifies a system of reliable, available, low-cost, and easy to use instruments; and recommends when these instruments should be used. The variables defined by AAPH fall into the six following categories:

- demographics
- cost per client care episode
- utilization of services
- level of functioning
- severity of symptoms
- client satisfaction.

CARF PE REQUIREMENTS FOR THE SIX PSYCHIATRIC PROGRAM TYPES

INPATIENT PSYCHIATRIC PROGRAM

- Movement into a less restrictive environment
- Readmission frequency by diagnosis
- Length of stay by diagnostic category
- Adverse incidents such as suicide attempts postdischarge

PARTIAL HOSPITALIZATION PROGRAM

- Movement into a less intensive level of care
- Increased levels of independence in day-to-day activities
- Movement toward social integration
- Decrease in frequency and duration of psychiatric hospitalizations

RESIDENTIAL TREATMENT PROGRAM

- Movement toward social integration
- Reduction of frequency and duration of psychiatric hospitalization
- Movement to a more independent vocational environment
- Movement to a more independent residential environment
- Length of stay norms by diagnosis
- Identification of the characteristics of persons served and prognosis for successful program completion

COMMUNITY HOUSING PROGRAMS

- Movement toward social integration

- Reduction of frequency and duration of psychiatric hospitalization

- Movement to a more independent residential environment

- Movement to a more independent vocational environment

OUTPATIENT THERAPY PROGRAMS

- Increased level of psychological functioning

- Increased self-esteem of person served

- Increased participation in community activities

EMERGENCY OR CRISIS INTERVENTION PROGRAM

- Referral to the least restrictive, appropriate alternative

- Reduction of hospital-bed days

- Reduction of critical incidents

- Minimization of inappropriate referrals

- Reduction of reported program interventions

As one easily can see, there are definite similarities in the program objectives and PE requirements for the different levels of psychiatric rehabilitation programs. AAPH[194] offers some excellent recommendations on appropriate outcome measures for the ambulatory-based mental health programs. Outcome measures for psychiatric programs tend to fall into the following categories:

- living status and community adjustment

- functional independence

- psychosocial adjustment

- vocational adjustment

- recidivism and resource utilization

- client/patient satisfaction.

Goal Attainment Scales (GAS)[199] have been a frequently used approach to outcome measurement in psychiatric rehabilitation programs. GAS customizes the outcome goal or expectation to individual clients and then measures their performance against that goal for each dimension of performance and behavior.

OUTCOME MEASURES

The outcome measures of level of functioning recommended by AAPH include:

- BASIS-32[202] (a clinician and client self-report measure)

- SF-36 (discussed previously under outpatient medical rehabilitation)

- Global Assessment of Functioning[195] (developed by the American Psychiatric Association)

- FACES III[206] (a level of functioning measure for children and adolescents)

- KATZ Activities of Daily Living[31] and Lawton/Brody IADL Scale[201] (level of function measures for geriatric patients)

- Mini Mental State Exam[198] and the Geriatric Depression Scale[207] (measures of severity of symptoms for geriatric patients).

In addition to the outcome measures recommended by AAPH, one should also consider the following standardized instruments: Brief Follow-Up Scale, Housing Scale, Social Functioning Scale, Brief Psychiatric Rating Scale, and General Health Questionnaire. For further information about these outcome measures the reader should contact the AAPH Outcomes Project (703) 836-2274, and the Center for Psychiatric Rehabilitation at Boston University (930 Commonwealth Avenue, Boston, MA 02215; 617-353-3549) and the Clarke Institute of Psychiatry of Toronto.(250 College Street, Toronto, Canada MST 1R8; 416-979-2221).

Galvin Andrews and colleagues have reviewed 95 outcome measures for their psychometric properties, reliability, validity, and suitability for various mental health settings. The measures fall into the categories of broad-spectrum symptom measures (18), measures of functioning (20), quality of life measures (17), measures of family burden (5), measures of satisfaction with services (8), and multidimensional measures (27). In order to be selected, the measures must meet minimal criteria for applicability, practicality, reliability, validity, and sensitivity to change.

A task force of measurement experts has recommended five measures as most suitable for mental health outcomes measurement. Three of these are brief, multidimensional self-report measures (Behaviour and Symptom Identification Scale, Mental Health Inventory, and Medical Outcomes Study Short Form 36) and two are brief clinical rating scales (Health of the Nation Outcome Scale, and Role of Functioning Scale), which are described briefly below. (The report of the task force was authored by G. Andrews, L. Peters, and M. Teeson and was entitled, *The Measurement of Consumer Outcomes in Mental Health: A Report to the National Mental Health Information Strategy Committee* and is available from Clinical Research Unity for Anxiety Disorders, Sydney, Australia.)

BEHAVIOUR AND SYMPTOM IDENTIFICATION SCALE (BASIS)

BASIS is a 32-item scale that can be administered by an interviewer or used as a patient self-report measure. It takes approximately 20 to 30 minutes to complete and emphasizes the patient's perspective on relation to self and others, daily living and role function, depression and anxiety, impulsive and addictive behavior, and psychosis. Given the brevity and ease of administration, the BASIS appears to be a suitable outcome measure for inpatient psychiatric care. BASIS has acceptable internal consistency of items, excellent test–retest reliability over a 2- or 3-day period, and adequate criterion-related and construct validity.

MENTAL HEALTH INVENTORY (MHI)

The MHI was designed to measure general psychological distress and well-being in the RAND Health Insurance Experiment. It is a 38-item, self-report measure covering five dimensions:

- anxiety

- depression

- loss of behavioral and emotional control

- general positive affect

- emotional ties.

These are rated for their frequency of occurrence on a 6-point scale. The psychometric properties of the MHI have been well tested and are satisfactory, with excellent internal consistency, and adequate content and construct validity. A brief version (MHI-5) of the instrument also has been developed.

MEDICAL OUTCOMES STUDY SHORT FORM (SF 36)

The SF-36, described earlier, is a 36-item self-administered measure of health-related quality of life that assesses psychiatric symptoms, functioning, and quality of life. The SF-36 takes only 5 to 10 minutes to complete and has been found to be an excellent predictor of future health care usage. Three of the 8 domains contained in the SF-36 focus on emotional role limitations, mental health, and social functioning. Extensive psychometric studies have been done on the SF-36, with demonstrated reliability, validity, and interclass and interitem analyses. The SF-36 has the advantage of allowing comparisons between mental health consumers and physical health consumers.

HEALTH OF THE NATION OUTCOME SCALES (HNOS)

HoNOS was developed in response to mental health targets set up by the UK Department of Health to significantly improve the health and social functioning of mentally ill people. It is a set of 12 scales that are completed by a trained mental health worker with input from the patient. The 12 scales cover the following:

- aggressive or disruptive behavior

- suicidal thoughts and serious injurious behavior

- health or social problems associated with alcohol and drug use

- memory problems

- orientation and understanding

- physical disorders

- mood disturbances

- hallucinations and delusions and other mental and behavior problems

- social relationships

- housing

- recreation

- finance

- overall severity of functional disability.

Training on the use of the scales is required. HoNOS emphasis is on patients with psychotic illnesses, and it may not be suitable for other psychiatric disorders. The psychometric properties, reliability, validity, and sensitivity to measure small increments of improvement currently are being evaluated.

ROLE OF FUNCTIONING (RFS)

The RFS was developed to measure level of functioning of mental health patients on a statewide basis in Georgia, in 1984. It is rated on a 7-point scale and has four domains:

- work

- independent living and self-care

- immediate social network

- extended social network.

It provides a Global Role Functioning Index, with excellent internal consistency, adequate test–retest and interrater reliability, and adequate construct and criterion-related validity. It has not been demonstrated to be sensitive to measure change as yet.

SPECIFIC LEVEL OF FUNCTIONING SCALE (SLOF)

The SLOF is a 43-item inventory rated on a 5-point Likert-type scale that assesses functioning on six subscales:

- physical functioning

- personal care skills

- interpersonal relationships

- social acceptability

- activities

- work skills.

SLOF appears to be a good measure of functional skills for severely mentally ill patients, but has questionable reliability, validity, and measurement properties.

The measurement task force did not find any adequate measures of quality of life, burden of care, or satisfaction with services that meet acceptable measurement criteria and are suitable to measure mental health outcomes across settings. Extreme caution should be exercised when using self-report patient measures as they may be susceptible to certain response sets (i.e., the tendency for patients to respond in certain ways depending on their mood, attention span, emotional distress, family problems, finances, and many other temporal factors). Outcome measures in mental health should focus more on the functional outcomes and not so much on symptom reduction, which may or may not impact the individual's ability to function independently in society. The main emphasis of outcomes in mental health should be on handicap-related issues and societal disadvantage suffered as a result of the impairment and mental health disability. Some of the global cross-sectional outcome measures like the RFS or GAF may provide some general clinical and functional outcomes across impairment groups, but may not be sensitive to the unique clinical aspects of any one mental disorder. Therefore, a combination of global outcome measures and impairment-specific measures usually is recommended. Global measures of functioning seem to be related to life satisfaction, while specific skill ratings by observers do not show this relationship.

MENTAL HEALTH STATISTICS PROGRAM (MHSIP)

In an attempt to develop a customer-oriented mental health report card, several task forces have been established under the auspices of the MHSIP program to outline measurement construction criteria, background, definitions of expected outcomes, and proposed report card domains. The project, which is now in phase III, will develop recommendations for specific indicators and measures to be pilot tested in a variety of psychiatric settings. The primary indicators can be categorized into

- appropriateness
- access
- efficiency
- adequacy
- effectiveness
- customer satisfaction.

The mental health performance indices may parallel the Health Plan Employer Data and Information Set (HEDIS) program used to evaluated managed care companies. For further information, contact Vijay Ganju, Ph.D., Chair, MHSIP Report Card Task Force, Texas Department of Mental Health.

HAND REHABILITATION PROGRAMS

The American Society of Hand Therapists (ASHT) is developing a database and evaluation tools called the UE Net[68,69], which stands for Upper Extremity Network. The software and methodology for the database are being developed by Rehabilitation Technology Works (RTW) in San Bernardino, CA, and the Greenleaf Medical Systems (GMS) of Palo Alto, CA. The UE Net will use standardized outcome measures that follow the ASHT Clinical Assessment Recommendations and the ASHT Splint Classification System. UE Net is expected to interact with clinical systems such as EVAL, EXOS, Dexter, Henley, and NK to provide for automated documentation, progress reporting, and billing functions. For more information contact Jean Casanova, Project Manager, by telephone at (414) 789-9943 or by mail at 17790 Marseille Drive, Broadfield, WI 53045-5020.

HOME HEALTH PROGRAMS

Home health programs and providers have become increasingly concerned about outcome measures and comparative performance with other providers. The Health Care Financing Administration (HCFA) has been working with the National Association for Home Care (NAHC),[74] in collaboration with the Centers for Health Policy and Research at the University of Colorado, to establish a national database and benchmark performance indices for home health. They will soon begin recruiting about 50 home health agencies to participate in a National Medicare QA Demonstration Project. For more information, contact Kathryn Crisler, at the Centers for Health Policy and Services Research, by telephone at (303) 756-8350 or by mail at 1355 South Colorado Blvd., Suite 306, Denver, CO 80222.

VHA NORTH CENTRAL PATIENT OUTCOMES SURVEY

A group of home health agencies from the Voluntary Hospital Association (VHA) of North America, 77 based in Minneapolis, is working to develop benchmark performance indices and an outcome data collection system for certain diagnoses. The group has developed eight outcome areas:

- medication compliance

- physiological stability

- control of risk factors

- knowledge of disease process

- level of function (ADL, IADL, and environmental safety)

- coping

- treatment and procedures

- social support.

The group has been focusing its development on outcome measures for the high-volume and high-risk home care populations: fractured hips, congestive heart failure, stroke, emphysema or Chronic Obstructive Pulmonary Disease (COPD), and diabetes. For more information, contact the VHA Task Force, Minneapolis, MN (3600 West 80 Street, Suite 550, Minneapolis, MN 55431; 612-896-3424).

HOME CARE DATA SYSTEMS

Home Care Data Systems[71] is a computerized reference database of outcomes for home health providers that provides a standardized system of collecting and reporting outcomes and a PC-based software program (for DOS). The home care component is available, and other components for home infusion therapy, durable medical equipment, and hospice care will be available in the future. Participating agencies pay an initial fee to join, plus data processing fees for monthly data submission. Agencies can collect their outcome data via paper and pencil abstract or computer software program, and submit their data to the reference database via diskette or modem. Agencies are expected to receive quarterly and annual reports with comparative national statistics. There is no information currently available on the reliability, validity, or psychometric properties of the proposed outcome measures. For more information, contact Kathy Morgan, HomeCare Education Specialists, Johnson City, TN at (615) 926-6992.

OUTCOME CONCEPT SYSTEMS, INC. (OCS)

Another example of a commercially available outcome measurement system for home health agencies is offered by OCS[75], based in Gig Harbor, WA. The system consists of outcome measurement and documentation. The costs of the PC-based software are between $5,000 and $10,000, depending on the size of the agency. At the present time there is no reference database, but one may be created in the near future. There is no information currently available on the reliability, validity, or psychometric properties of the proposed outcome measures. For more information, contact OCS at (206) 858-7492 or write to: Outcome Concept Systems, Inc., 12804 47th Ave., NW, Gig Harbor, WA 98332.

HEALTH STATUS QUESTIONNAIRE (HSQ)

The Health Status Questionnaire[70], developed by the Health Outcomes Institute, is designed to measure overall functional status, well-being, and risk of depression in adults. The tool has been used in a variety of settings, regardless of diagnosis, and assesses eight specific health attributes in three major health dimensions:

- overall evaluation of health (general health perception)

- functional status (physical and social functioning, role limitations)

- well-being (pain, mental health, energy/fatigue).

The HSQ, which is very similar to the SF-36 described earlier, has established reliability, validity, and measurement properties. However, as with the SF-36, the HSQ may not be well suited for the geriatric disabled. For more information on the HSQ, contact the Health Outcomes Institute at (612) 858-9188 or write to Health Outcomes Institute, 2001 Killebrew Dr., Suite 122, Bloomington, MN 55425.

UDSMR[SM] HOME HEALTH OUTCOME MEASURES

The Uniform Data System for Medical Rehabilitation[76] has begun a pilot study to develop outcome measures and a national database for home care patients receiving rehabilitation services. Sixteen home health agencies are participating in the study. Results are pending completion of the data analysis and a report was due March 1, 1996. UD$_{MR}$[SM] has added a number of items to the FIM[SM], including the FASQ, and is assessing functional outcomes for various impairment groups and services provided. Additionally, they are collecting units of service (measured in minutes) for each discipline. There currently are 100 records abstracted from 16 home health agencies. For more information, contact UDS_{MR}^{SM} at (716) 829-2076 or write to: USD_{MR}^{SM}, 232 Parker Hall, State University of New York at Buffalo, 3435 Main St., Buffalo, NY 14214-3007.

FORMATIONS IN HEALTH CARE — HOME HEALTH CARE OUTCOME SCALE

Formations in Health Care[72] also is developing an outcome system for home health, using many of the indicators from the LADS, Neuro Rehabilitation, Orthopedic Outpatient, and MOS outcome systems. There are over 500 records abstracted from 9 participating home health agencies in the database. Reliability and validity results are pending completion of the field test. For more information, contact Formations in Health Care at (312) 849-4200. ∎

10. METHODS OF PRESENTING AND REPORTING OUTCOME RESULTS

Outcome information is needed by program managers, administrators, governing bodies, third party payers, referring professionals and agencies, potential consumers and purchasers of services, and the community. Those persons and organizations that are in a position to make decisions and facilitate change or improve performance and outcome should have access to outcome information[187] and it should be presented in a manner that is clear, concise, timely, understandable, and relevant. Different methods of providing feedback information should be used for different audiences. The more commonly used methods of presenting information include statistics, graphs, matrices, narrative descriptions, and client satisfaction comments as described in the following section.

STATISTICS

Several methods are available for collecting and summarizing statistical data. Two commonly used methods are criteria measures and improvement measures.[120]

CRITERIA MEASURES

The criteria measure identifies in absolute terms the specific outcome (either at discharge or follow-up) desired. Criteria-oriented measures usually are expressed in terms of the percentage of clients who have reached a previously established level of performance by a specific point in time. Some[135,187] claim that the advantage of using a criteria measure is that the information presented has more meaning and a greater likelihood of impact on changing or modifying client programs and outcomes. Criteria measures can be easy to interpret.

IMPROVEMENT MEASURES

The improvement measure assesses change in a client's functional abilities or limitations over time. An improvement measure can provide information on the amount of change and also describe the functional outcome of clients. One investigator[106] compared estimates of outcomes with actual patient records and follow-up interviews. In another study[136], the authors found evidence that progress gained through rehabilitation was retained after discharge and that the functional level typically was higher at follow-up.

The use of criteria-oriented measures (percentages) versus improvement measures (amount of gain) is still an area of considerable controversy. The use of improvement measures allows evaluators to describe the functional level of the client upon entry into the program, amount of functional gains made in the program as well as after discharge, and the final functional level attained by the client at follow-up. However, the evaluator must remember that the rating scale used in the functional assessment instrument may not approximate the characteristics of a true interval scale, making the use of mean and standard deviation statistics inappropriate. Care must be taken in the development and interpretation of the scale and of reliability and validity data. Rasch and factor analyses can shed light on the scaling properties, precision, unidimensionality, item weighting, and fit of the items in the inventory or major factors, and also can transform ratings on an ordinal scale to an interval scale to allow appropriate parametric statistics (e.g., gain score, averages, means, standard deviations) to be applied. For most evaluators, the advantages of using improvement measures far outweigh those for alternative methods of summarizing data, and the disadvantages are minimal.

GRAPHS

Graphs can be used to display functional improvements and can add perceptual clarity to the statistics as reviewers are given a visual presentation of the data. Histograms (bar graphs) and polygrams (line graphs) should be used whenever possible to display functional outcome data. Figure 10, based on hypothetical data, provides an example of a histogram that can be used to display means scores on admission, discharge, and follow-up for a number of different self-care items.

MATRICES

Another useful technique for displaying functional outcome data is through the use of a matrix. The matrix in Figure 11 displays the admission and discharge scores for 26 stroke patients on the item of dressing. For example, of those patients who had a score of 2 at admission, two had a discharge score of 2, 11 a discharge score of 3, and four a discharge score of 4. The two irregular diagonal lines separate those who improved from those who stayed the same.

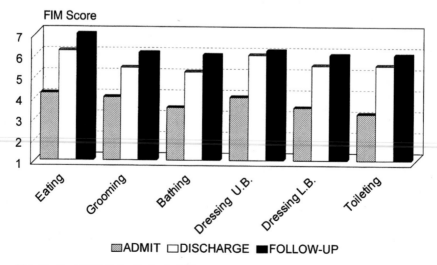

FIGURE 10

Average FIM Self Care - Stroke

ADMIT   DISCHARGE   FOLLOW-UP

Hypothetical UDS Data, first admissions

FIGURE 11.

Discharge Score

		1	2	3	4
	4	0	0	0	1
Admission Score	3	0	1	2	1
	2	0	2	11	4
	1	1	2	1	0

NARRATIVE DESCRIPTIONS

Clinical and management staff often are more interested in a narrative description or summary of results than they are in actual statistics, graphs, or matrices. Quantifiable data or scores are needed for statistical or comparison purposes, while a description of abilities is needed for more practical and clinical applications. Narrative descriptions should accompany outcome data whenever possible because they help to interpret the data and are understood more easily by staff. Outcome scales should be constructed so they are clinically relevant and scores can easily be translated back into clinical terms.

CLIENT SATISFACTION COMMENTS

The structured interview and functional status rating instrument should encourage comments. Such comments from former clients, family members, or significant others can supplement or clarify functional status ratings. Additionally, it is advisable to query former clients and family members about their satisfaction with the rehabilitation program and services and to solicit any concerns they may have. Because this type of information often is difficult to quantify, comments usually are reported separately from other outcome data. One technique is to separate positive and negative comments and to provide specific departments with feedback pertinent to their areas only. The evaluator consequently avoids creating resentment among staff members for sharing confidential and potentially threatening negative information. Also recommended, however, is a built-in accountability system to respond to comments and accusations from former clients and family members. ■

11. ANALYZING FINDINGS, DEVELOPING ACTION PLANS, AND CONDUCTING FOLLOW-UP

Once a quality and outcome evaluation system has been implemented, measures have been selected, data analysis has been completed, and results begin to become available, there are a number of important steps that should be taken in analyzing and interpreting findings, developing action plans, and conducting follow-up on the results of corrective actions or changes implemented. These important steps include:

- team review

- trend or pattern analysis

- comparison of functional and medical status on admission and discharge

- comparisons with external reference groups and regional or national data

- consideration of extraneous variables

- development of an executive summary

- development of action-oriented recommendations

- assignment of responsible parties

- follow-up review.

TEAM REVIEW

The entire treatment team should be involved in developing, implementing, and analyzing outcome evaluation results. Once results are generated, they should be reviewed by the entire team to identify problem areas, trends, possible extraneous variables and explanations, recommendations, and action plans. Although the team may not be the final decision-making body, its members often can add useful insight into the interpretation of findings. The program director or manager should first review and discuss the results with the clinical team before making recommendations to management. Once the reports have been reviewed by the treating team, they can be passed on to other review committees with comments and recommendations.

TRENDS

Looking for trends in outcome evaluation findings between quarters or perhaps across several years may provide important information. Significant changes may be detected in patient characteristics or needs, time from onset to admission, length or duration of treatment, and other factors that may require program modification. One also should determine if past actions taken have been effective in resolving problems. This is one extremely important step that often is overlooked.

FUNCTIONAL LEVELS ON ADMISSION AND DISCHARGE

It is important to describe the functional level of patients upon admission, the gains made in the program as well as after discharge, and the final functional status at follow-up. Clients in one quarter may be more or less impaired than during previous quarters, affecting both their potential for improvement and the final outcome.

COMPARISON WITH NATIONAL AND REGIONAL DATA

Many management decisions require the availability of comparable data from other facilities. We need to look toward standardization and uniformity of evaluation and management information systems to allow comparisons among facilities and regions. Several states have organized datasharing activities. Two basic methods of data sharing are used:

- annual surveys providing aggregate or summarized results

- reporting data about individual clients.

These surveys provide statistical information needed to support or oppose pertinent legislation and regulations and also provide participating facilities with comparative data that can be used for planning and management purposes. Some trade and state rehabilitation associations, including AOTA, provide annual surveys or reference databases to allow providers to compare their performance against similar providers. Care should be taken to ensure that equitable comparisons are made and that the database is severity adjusted.

On the national level, many of the data management services described in Section VII provide comparative regional and national outcome information. Sometimes comparative regional and national figures are published in the professional journals. There usually is a substantial time lag (12–24 months) before such comparative results get published. This generally is not frequent enough for a provider to make timely and effective improvements in quality and outcome.

CONSIDERATION OF EXTRANEOUS VARIABLES AND EXPLANATIONS

There often are very simple explanations for less than desirable patient and program outcomes, such as program interruptions, medical complications, placement problems, or lack of family support and patient motivation. Several studies[137,138,151] have shown that therapists consistently rate patients higher than do patients themselves. Nurses tend to rate patients as being at lower levels of functioning than do therapists, and families often tend to underestimate patients' ability to do things for themselves. Nurses, facing time and caseload pressures, have less time to allow patients to complete tasks such as dressing themselves, and must provide adequate supervision for safety reasons. Therapists observe the patients in a structured setting, without some of these pressures and constraints, and tend to rate the patient at higher functional levels. A patient's anxiety, depression, and level of satisfaction with adjustment may taint his or her functional status rating. Family members often are inclined to provide assistance to a patient who is having difficulty with an activity or taking too long, rather than watch his or her struggle. The clinical team needs to be given the opportunity to explain any undesirable or unexpected variance in the outcomes. These explanations and assumptions can be tested and validated later.

EXECUTIVE SUMMARY

A narrative executive summary should accompany outcome evaluation reports. The executive summary can be used to highlight the findings and bring out important comparisons. For example:

> Patients appeared to be just as impaired on admission as in previous quarters and showed more improvement from admission to discharge. In the area of self-care, on the average, patients required minimal assistance on admission, the goal was modified independence, and at discharge patients still required some supervision, extra time, or assistive devices. Compared to national figures, our patients were more impaired on admission and made 25 percent more progress during rehabilitation than patients in other facilities.

RECOMMENDATIONS

Each problem area should be clearly identified, with explanations, comments, and recommendations. Here are some examples:

Outcome Indicator/ Program Objective	Threshold	Results	Recommendations
Increase Self-Care Skills (Stroke) Average FIM^{SM} gain on 6 self-care items from admission to discharge	1.4	1.2	Review cases failing to meet program threshold to determine appropriateness of OT treatment, plan type and intensity of services provided, clinical expertise of staff, skill mix and use of group treatment. Review acuity and severity of cases.
Maintain Functional Gains Percent of patients who maintain or improve FIM^{SM} scores after discharge	80%	70%	Investigate functional deterioration postdischarge, identify poor performance areas, and ensure patients are receiving appropriate follow-up care and therapy.

RESPONSIBLE PARTIES

The disciplines and responsible parties for overseeing and carrying out various recommendations should be identified.

FOLLOW-UP

Each recommendation should be followed up to ensure that actions taken have been effective in addressing the issue. Contingency plans should be developed if intended corrective actions were not effective in improving results. This analysis should be used in the redesign of programs and services. ■

IV.
CONCLUSION

12. FUTURE TRENDS AND DIRECTIONS

In this last section, anticipated future trends and directions in health care as they may impact the occupational therapy practitioner in different care settings are discussed. Decisions about access, entitlements, covered benefits, cost-benefits or expected return on certain high-cost procedures, and general public health education and prevention are likely to become the center stage of political debates and public health policy. Third party payers, including the federal government, are anxious to develop health care report cards to profile and compare providers. It is therefore likely there will be more emphasis placed on outcomes and cost-effectiveness, effective quality improvement and management techniques, opportunities to help educate customer groups and define appropriate outcomes to be expected from rehabilitation efforts, projected cost savings in terms of future health care usage, and prevention of subsequent medical complications.

PRICE VERSUS QUALITY AND OUTCOME CONSIDERATIONS

Third party payers, particularly managed care organizations and workers' compensation carriers, have become increasingly concerned with long-term outcomes, total case costs, and future health care usage. Although, for the moment, price appears to be the single most important determinant in the selection and utilization of providers, these third party payers and managed care organizations will begin to pay much more attention to quality and outcome issues to avoid unnecessary risk and liability exposure that may result from denied or restricted access to care. A number of class action suits have recently been filed against the nation's largest managed care companies. The main issue focuses around denied access to reasonable and medically necessary services. Several of these cases have recently settled and are likely to force managed care entities to pay more attention to quality and outcome measures in addition to cost. Therefore, in the near future, payers will begin to demand outcome data, government will be asking for outcome data, and employers will be looking for value. Occupational therapy practitioners must be prepared to provide this type of quality and outcome data and to demonstrate the cost-effectiveness and benefits of the services they provide.

Most managed care companies are not particularly knowledgeable in the areas of quality and outcome management, although some of the older, more sophisticated managed care organizations (MCOs) have developed elaborate provider profile and tracking systems that include some outcome measures. The managed care companies will set up systems to continually monitor the quality, outcome, client satisfaction, and undesirable consequences of care for various providers. Therefore, there is a short window of opportunity for occupational therapy providers to help define accreditation standards, quality and outcome measures, and design evaluation systems so they can influence what criteria are used by managed care entities, governmental agencies, and employers in evaluating providers. Providers should be prepared to address the outcome expectations of managed care entities: qualifications and expertise of providers, injury/reinjury prevention, medical complications, long-term outcomes, total case costs, and reduction of future health care usage.

USING QUALITY AND OUTCOME RESULTS IN MANAGED CARE CONTRACT NEGOTIATIONS

Many providers are using their outcome and quality results in contract negotiations with managed care entities. Full functional recovery may not be the primary outcome expectation of most managed care entities. Instead, many MCOs want to make coverage and payment decisions based on generally acceptable outcomes at the least cost. Occupational therapy practitioners, therefore, must be willing to negotiate with MCOs based on compromise outcomes that may be minimally acceptable to the patient, family, and MCO. If health care resources are managed effectively, and the most cost-effective treatment techniques are provided, what types of outcome are reasonable at a given price? Programs must be able to respond with meaningful data for various customer groups in order to answer the question, "What can I expect to get for my health care dollars?" Part of the practitioner's role is to educate various consumer groups on what minimally acceptable outcomes should be and the long-term cost savings of various programs. The burden of proof falls on the provider. Otherwise, managed care organizations will expect the same intensity of service, quality, and outcome at a lower price, which may not be possible.

PROVIDER NETWORKING AND SERVICE INTEGRATION

Since there is a trend toward bundling of services and "one-stop shopping," many providers have formed coalitions and networks to contract with MCOs and other third party payers. Occupational therapy practitioners can gain contracting advantages through affiliations and networks with other practitioners, disciplines, and care settings. The larger MCOs are not interested in negotiating contracts with small independent providers or provider systems. They want to be able to ensure appropriate access to required medical and mental health services, at the lowest possible cost, through a coordinated continuum of care network. Under a capitated environment, providers will be forced to develop alliances with all aspects of the continuum of care. The ability to effectively manage cases across the continuum becomes essential for survival.

REENGINEERING THE DELIVERY SYSTEM

In order to provide more cost-effective services and acceptable outcomes at the lowest cost and with the least amount of resource utilization, providers must begin to think of innovative approaches to treatment. This may involve the increased utilization of group treatment, paraprofessionals and aides, physician extenders, and less intensive, lower cost treatment settings. In 1991, based on a survey of 300 rehabilitation providers[176], approximately 25 percent of OT treatment in acute inpatient rehabilitation and subacute settings and 30% of outpatient rehabilitation were provided in groups of 3 or more patients. Today, it is estimated that as much as 30 percent of OT in acute rehabilitation, 50 percent in subacute, and 40 percent in outpatient rehabilitation is provided in groups, according to a survey by the American Rehabilitation Association (1994).[161] Some of these group sessions are led by OTRs in combination with aides, assistants, and other disciplines. Studies must be done within each practice setting to ensure the appropriate utilization of groups along with the best possible outcomes. The effectiveness of group treatment must be continuously monitored. Selection criteria and objectives for each group should be established. There also is a trend toward the use of paraprofessionals, aides, and assistants who are cross-trained among a number of disciplines (e.g., PT, OT, ST, and RN). There will be a continued need for collaboration among disciplines to develop less costly multiskilled personnel.

The focus of occupational therapy treatment will shift to providing what is absolutely essential to enable a patient to move to the least costly or restrictive treatment environment. The appropriateness of various OT treatment goals will be based on essential aspects of a patient's recovery and skills (performance areas) that must be accomplished at each stage of the continuum to ensure a safe transition into the next level of care. The impact of these changes in the delivery system on costs, outcomes, quality of care, and customer satisfaction must be carefully evaluated.

RATIONING AND ELIGIBILITY REQUIREMENTS

Given the health care reform effort and the influence of managed care, priorities and eligibility requirements for given procedures and treatment settings are likely to be based on expected outcome, prognosis, cost, and return on investment. As seniors sign over their Medicare benefits to MCOs, their access to traditional health care services will become more restrictive because the MCOs will have strong financial incentives to minimize health care utilization as they do with the younger, healthier populations. The irony is that seniors are led to believe they will have expanded benefits and access to care under a MCO senior plan. The new Medicare reform proposals may provide more options for seniors with better controls to ensure access to appropriate care. Workers' compensation carriers will only invest in treatment and procedures with proven outcomes (short and long term). In many regions of the country, both Medicare and Medicaid managed care options are more prevalent. More and more, authorization, coverage, and payment decisions will be based on outcome results.

MERGERS, ACQUISITIONS, AND AGGRESSIVE MARKETING

Occupational therapy practitioners will continue to see mergers and acquisitions of health care providers and delivery systems in attempts to reposition themselves for regional and national contracting. These larger entities will continue aggressive marketing programs to promote increased access to their services. Occupational therapy practitioners must become skilled marketers and be able to effectively promote and sell their services. Demonstrated quality, outcome, and cost-effectiveness will become prerequisites for participation in a large health care system. At the same time, we are likely to see a consolidation of MCOs due to buy-outs, bankruptcy, federal investigation, and regulation. The role of the surviving MCOs will shift to more emphasis on data analysis, information systems technology and long-term fund development. The providers will then assume the risk of managing health care resources and will make changes based on feedback from their own internal information systems and data from MCOs to control costs. This implies better clinical resource management, based in part on best practices, clinical pathways, and an effective case management system of care across the continuum. ■

REFERENCES

For more detailed information on outcome measures for specific practice settings, programs, and impairment groups the reader is referred to the following references, which have been subdivided into 20 categories for fast and easy reference.

ACCREDITATION AGENCIES AND STANDARDS

1   Accreditation Council on Services for People with Disabilities. (1993). *Outcomes-based performance measures.* Landover, MD: Accreditation Council on Services for People with Disabilities.

2   *Accreditation manual for hospitals.* (1995). Oakbrook Terrace, IL: Joint Commission on Accreditation of Healthcare Organizations.

3   Commission on Accreditation of Rehabilitation Facilities. (1995, January). *1995 Standards for medical rehabilitation.* Tuscon, AZ: Author.

4   Joint Commission on Accreditation of Healthcare Organizations. (1995). *1995 Survey protocol for subacute programs.* Oakbrook, IL: Author.

5   Joint Commission on Accreditation of Healthcare Organizations. (1994). *The measurement mandate: On the road to performance improvement in health care.* Oakbrook Terrace, IL: Author.

BRAIN INJURY REHABILITATION OUTCOME MEASURES

6   Cope, D.N., & Hall, K. (1982). Head injury rehabilitation: Benefits of early intervention. *Archives of Physical Medicine and Rehabilitation, 82,* 433–437.

7   Diller, L., & Ben-Yishay, Y. (1987). Analyzing rehabilitation outcomes of persons with head injury. In M.J. Fuhrer (Ed.), *Rehabilitation outcomes: Analysis and measurement.* Baltimore, MD: Brookes Publishing.

8   Hall, K. (1992). Overview of functional assessment scales in brain injury rehabilitation. *NeuroRehabilitation: An Interdisciplinary Journal, 2*(4), 98–113.

9   Hall, K. et al. (1993). Characteristics and comparisons of functional assessment indices: Disability Rating Scale, Functional Independence Measure, and the Functional Assessment Measure. *Journal of Head Trauma Rehabilitation, 8*(2), 60–74.

10 Jennette, B., & Bond, M. (1975). Assessment of outcome after severe brain damage: A practical scale. *Lancet, 1,* 480–484.

11 Johnston, M.V., & Hall, K. (1994). Outcome evaluation in traumatic brain injury rehabilitation. *Archives of Physical Medicine and Rehabilitation, 75* (12-S).

12   Malkmus, D. (1979). Cognitive assessment and goal setting: The Rancho Levels of Cognitive Function (LCFS). In *Rehabilitation of Head Injured Adults: Comprehensive Management.* Downey, CA: Rancho Los Amigos Hospital.

13   McDowel, I., & Newell, C. (1987). *Measuring health: A guide to rating scales and questionnaires.* New York: Oxford University Press.

14   Rappaport, M., Hall, K., Hopkins, K. et al. (1982). Disability Rating Scale for severe head trauma: Coma to community. *Archives of Physical Medicine and Rehabilitation, 63,* 118–123.

15   Teasdale, G., & Jennette, B. (1975). Assessment of coma and impaired consciousness: A practical scale. *Lancet, 1,* 480–484.

16   Willer, B. et al. (1993). Assessment of community integration following traumatic brain injury. *Journal of Head Trauma Rehabilitation, 8*(2), 75–87.

COMMUNITY REENTRY AND LIVING OUTCOME MEASURES

17   Cole, J.R., Coper, D.N., & Cervelli, L. (1985). Rehabilitation of the severely brain-injured patient: A community-based low-cost model program. *Archives of Physical Medicine and Rehabilitation, 66,* 38–40.

18   Fuhrer, M.J., Rossi, L.D., Gerken, L. et al. (1990). Relationships between independent living centers and medical rehabilitation programs. *Archives of Physical Medicine and Rehabilitation, 71,* 519–522.

19   Nosek, M. (1987). Outcome analysis in independent living. In M.J. Fuhrer (Ed.), *Rehabilitation outcomes: Analysis and measurement.* Baltimore, MD: Brookes Publishing.

20   Nosek, M.A. (1984). *Relationships among measures of social independence, psychological independence, and functional abilities in adults with severe orthopedic impairments.* Doctoral dissertation, University of Texas.

21   Ross, H. (1980). The relationship between level and object relations and degree of autonomy in mothers and their daughters. *Dissertation Abstracts Inter., 41*(5), 1894A–1895A.

22   Wikerson, D., Weinhouse, S., & Jamero, P. (1982). *Independent living center evaluation: Washington State data system and data from the first year of Title VII.* Seattle, WA: University of Washington.

COMPREHENSIVE INPATIENT REHABILITATION OUTCOME MEASURES

23   Brown, M., Gordon, W., & Diller, W. Rehabilitation indicators. In A.S. Halpern & M.J. Fuhrer (Eds.), *Functional assessment in rehabilitation* (pp. 187–204). Baltimore, MD: Brookes Publishing.

24   Carey, R.G., & Posavac, E.J. (1978). Program evaluation of a physical medicine and rehabilitation unit: A new approach. *Archives of Physical Medicine and Rehabilitation, 59,* 330–337.

25   Forer, S. (1982). Functional assessment instrument in medical rehabilitation. *Journal of the Organization of Rehabilitation Evaluators, 2,* 29–41.

26   Harvey, R.F., & Jellinek, H.M. (1983). Patient profiles: Utilization in functional performance assessment. *Archives of Physical Medicine and Rehabilitation, 64,* 268–271.

27   Granger, C., Albrehct, G., & Hamilton, B. (1979). Outcome of comprehensive medical rehabilitation: Measurement of PULSES profile and Barthel. *Archives of Physical Medicine and Rehabilitation, 60,* 145–154.

28   Harvey, R., Silverstein, B. et al. (1992). Applying psychometric criteria to functional assessment in medical rehabilitation III: Construct validity and predicting level of care. *Archives of Physical Medicine and Rehabilitation, 73,* 887–892.

29   Iverson, I., Silbergerg, N., Stever, R., & Schoening, H. (1973). *The Revised Kenny Self Care Evaluation.* Minneapolis, MN: Sister Kenny Institute.

30   Jette, A. (1980). Functional status index: Reliability of a chronic disease evaluation instrument. *Archives of Physical Medicine and Rehabilitation, 61,* 395–401.

31   Katz, S., Ford, R.Q. et al. (1963). Studies of illness in the aged. The Index of ADL: A standardized measure of biological and psychological function. *JAMA, 185,* 914–919.

32   LORS II American Data System (LADS). (1991). Chicago, IL: Formations in Health Care.

33   Mahoney, F., & Barthel, D. (1965). Functional assessment: The Barthel Index. *MD State Medical Journal, 14,* 61–65.

34   Questad, K.A., Boltwood, M. et al. (1987). A comprehensive battery for the measurement of rehabilitation outcomes after major burns. In M.J. Fuhrer (Ed.), *Rehabilitation outcomes: Analysis and measurement.* Baltimore, MD: Brookes Publishing.

35   Rehabilitation Institute of Chicago. (September 1992). *Rehabilitation Institute of Chicago—Functional Assessment Scale version 3* (RIC–FAS III). Chicago, IL: Author.

36   Sarno, J., Sarno, M., & Levita, E. (1973). Functional life scale. *Archives of Physical Medicine and Rehabilitation, 54,* 214–220.

37   Silverstein, B., Fisher, W., Kilgore, K., Harley, P., & Harvey, R. (1992). Applying psychometric criteria to functional assessment in medical rehabilitation: II. Defining interval measures. *Archives of Physical Medicine and Rehabilitation, 73,* 507–517.

38   Susset, V., Vobecky, J., & Balck, R. (1979). Disability outcomes and self assessment of disabled persons: An analysis of 506 cases. *Archives of Physical Medicine and Rehabilitation, 60,* 50–56.

39   Uniform Data System for Medical Rehabilitation. (1993). *A Guide for the Uniform Data Set for Medical Rehabilitation (Adult FIM), version 4.0.* Buffalo, NY: State University of New York–Buffalo and the Center for Functional Assessment Research.

40   Wagner, K. (1987). Outcome analysis for comprehensive medical rehabilitation. In M.J. Fuhrer (Ed.), *Rehabilitation outcomes: Analysis and measurement.* Baltimore, MD: Brookes Publishing.

41   Williamson, J. (1971). Evaluating quality of patient care: Strategy relating outcome and process assessment. *JAMA, 218,* 564–569.

DATA MANAGEMENT SERVICES

42   Data Med Clinical Support Systems. (1993) *Computerized Healthcare Outcome Management: Assurance Rehabilitation and Long Term Care Systems.* Minneapolis, MN: Author.

43   Granger, C.V., Hamilton, B., & Forer, S. (1985). Development of a uniform national data system for medical rehabilitation (abstract). *Archives of Physical Medicine and Rehabilitation, 66,* 538–539.

44   Granger, C., & Hamilton B. (1994). The Uniform Data System for Medical Rehabilitation: Report of first admissions for 1992. *American Journal of Physical Medicine and Rehabilitation, 73*(1): 51–55.

45   Granger, C., Ottenbacher, K., & Fiedler, R. (1995). The Uniform Data System for Medical Rehabilitation: Report of first admissions for 1993. *American Journal of Physical Medicine and Rehabilitation, 74*(1), 62–66.

46   Harvey, R.F., & Jellinek, H.M. (1981). Functional performance assessment: A program approach. *Archives of Physical Medicine and Rehabilitation, 62,* 456–461.

47   *Home Care Data Systems.* (1995). Johnson City, TN: HomeCare Education Specialists.

48   Hospital Utilization Project of Pennsylvania. (1974). *Rehabilitation facility program procedure manual.* Pittsburgh, PA: Author.

49   *Indicator Management System (IM System).* (1995). Oakbrook Terrace, IL: Joint Commission on Accreditation of Healthcare Organizations.

50   Keith, R.A., & Breckenridge, K. (1985). Characteristics of patients from the Hospital Utilization Project data system: 1980–1982. *Archives of Physical Medicine and Rehabilitation, 66,* 768–772.

51   LORS III American Data System. (LADS). (1991). Chicago, IL: Formations in Healthcare, Inc. (312) 849–4200.

52   Medical Outcome System. (1994). Chicago, IL: Formations in Healthcare.

53   Posavac, E.J., & Carey, R.G. (1982, November–December). Using a level of function scale (LORS-II) to evaluate the success of inpatient rehabilitation programs. *Journal of Rehabilitation Nursing,* 17–19.

54   *Rehabilitation manager.* (1988). Chicago, IL: National Easter Seal Systems, (software release).

55   R/COM *Software for Rehabilitation Clinic Operation and Management.* (1983). Seattle, WA.

56   Upper Extremity Network (UE NET).(American Society of Hand Therapists Data Base). (1994). Chicago, IL: American Society of Hand Therapists.

EARLY INTERVENTION AND CHILD DEVELOPMENT OUTCOME MEASURES

57   Allen, D. (1987). Measuring rehabilitation outcomes for infants and young children: A family approach. In M.J. Fuhrer (Ed.), *Rehabilitation outcomes: Analysis and measurement* (pp. 185–195). Baltimore, MD: Brookes Publishing.

58   Affeck, G., McGrade, B., McQueeney, M., & Allen D. (1982). Promise of relationship-focused early intervention in developmental disabilities. *Journal of Special Education, 16,* 413–430.

59   Alexander, J., & Willems, E. (1981). Quality of life: Some measurement requirements. *Archives of Physical Medicine and Rehabilitation, 62,* 261–265.

60   Halpern, A.S. (1987). Outcome analysis for persons with mental retardation. In M.J. Fuhrer (Ed.), *Rehabilitation outcomes: Analysis and measurement.* Baltimore, MD: Brookes.

61 Halpern, R. (1984). Lack of effects for home-based early intervention? Some possible explanations. *American Journal of Orthopsychiatry, 54,* 33–42.

62 Loor, M., & McNair, D. (1982). *Profile of Mood States-B.* San Diego, CA: Education and Industrial Testing Service.

63 Newborg, J., Stock, J. et al. (1984). *The Battelle Developmental Inventory.* Allen, TX: DLM Teaching Resources.

64 Simeonsson, R., Cooper, D., & Scheneir, A. (1982). A review and analysis of the effectiveness of early education programs. *Pediatrics, 62,* 635–641.

65 Sparrow, S., Balla, D., & Cicchette, D. (1984). *Vineland Behavioral Scales.* Circle Pines, MN: American Guidance Service.

66 Waisbern, S. (1980). Parents' reaction after birth of a developmentally disabled child. *American Journal of Mental Deficiency, 84,* 345–351.

67 *WeeFIM: A Functional Independence Measure for pediatric rehabilitation ages 6 months to 7 years* (1993). Buffalo, NY: UDS$_{MR}$^{SM}, SUNY-Buffalo, and the Center for Functional Assessment Research.

HAND REHABILITATION OUTCOME MEASURES

68 Cohen, R. (1994, January–March). Strategies for positioning in the managed care market place. *Journal of Hand Therapy, 7*(1), 5–9.

69 *Upper Extremity Network (UE Net).* Chicago, IL: American Society of Hand Therapists.

HOME HEALTH OUTCOME MEASURES

70 *Health Status Questionnaire (HSQ).* (1991). Minneapolis, MN: Health Outcomes Institute.

71 *Home Care Data Systems.* (1995). Johnson City, TN: HomeCare Education Specialists.

72 *Home Health Care Outcome Scale.* (1995). Chicago, IL: Formations in Health Care.

73 Moore, A. (1993). Functional outcomes of patients with hip fractures in the home care setting. *Journal of Home Health Care Practice, 5*(4), 49–58.

74 National Association of Home Care. *Outcome-based quality improvement: A manual for home agencies on how to use outcomes.* (1995). Denver, CO: Centers for Health Policy and Services Research, University of Colorado.

75 *Outcome Concepts Systems, Inc. (OCS).* (1995). Gig Harbor, WA. (software documentation system).

76 *UDS$_{MR}$^{SM} Home Health Outcome Measures.* (1995). Buffalo, NY: UDS$_{MR}$^{SM}, SUNY-Buffalo, and the Center for Functional Assessment Research.

77 *VHA North Central Patient Outcomes Survey.* (1995). Minneapolis, MN: Voluntary Hospital Association (VHA) of North America Task Force.

OCCUPATIONAL REHABILITATION OUTCOME MEASURES

78 Hester, E, & Decelles, P. (1985). *The disability system: A dynamic analysis.* Topeka, KS: The Menninger Foundation.

79   Hood, L., & Downs, J. (1985). *Return-to-work: A literature review.* Topeka, KS: The Menninger Foundation.

80   King, P.M. (1993). Outcome analysis of work-hardening programs. *American Journal of Occupational Therapy, 4*(7), 595–603.

81   Muller, L. (1983). *Receipt of multiple benefits by disabled worker beneficiaries.* Washington, DC: U.S. Department of Health and Human Services, Social Security Administration.

82   *Occupational Outcome Scale.* (1995). Chicago, IL: Formations in Health Care.

83   *Work and Industrial Rehabilitation Evaluation (WIRE).* (1994). Bethesda, MD: AOTA.

OUTCOME EVALUATION

84   Forer, S.K. (1987). Outcome analysis for program service management. In M.J. Fuhrer (Ed.), *Rehabilitation outcomes: Analysis and measurement* (pp. 115–136). Baltimore, MD: Brookes Publishing.

85   Forer, S.K. (1991). *Product line management in the rehabilitation industry.* Washington, DC: National Association of Rehabilitation Facilities.

86   Forer, S.K., & Miller, L.S. (1980). Paraprofessional volunteers and the collection of program evaluation data. *Archives of Physical Medicine and Rehabilitation,61,* 490.

87   Formations in Health Care, Inc. (1995, May). *Outcomes across the continuum of care.* (Brochure and flyer). Chicago, IL: Author.

88   Fuhrer, M.J. (Ed.). (1987). *Rehabilitation outcomes: Analysis and measurement.* Baltimore, MD: Brooks Publishing.

89   Health Outcomes Institute. (1991). *Health Status Questionnaire (HSQ).* Bloomington, MN: Author.

90   Jenkins, C., Jono, R., Stanton, B., & Stroupp-Benham, C. (1990). The measurement of health-related quality of life: Major dimensions identified by factor analysis. *Social Science and Medicine, 31*(8), 925–931.

91   Jette, D., & Downing, J. (1994). Health status of individuals entering a cardiac rehabilitation program as measured by the Medical Outcomes Study 36 item short-form inventory. *Physical Therapy, 74*(6), 521–527.

92   Johnston, M., Wilkerson, D., & Maney, M. (1993). Evaluation of the quality and outcomes of medical rehabilitation programs. In J.A. Delisa (Ed.), *Rehabilitation medicine: Principles and practice* (pp. 240–268). Philadelphia, PA: Lippincott.

93   LaRocca, N.G. (1987). Analyzing outcomes in the care of persons with multiple sclerosis. In M.J. Fuhrer (Ed.), *Rehabilitation outcomes: Analysis and measurement.* Baltimore, MD: Brookes Publishing.

94   McHorney, C., Ware, J., & Raczek, A. (1993). The MOS 36 item Short-Form Health Survey (SF-36): II. Psychometric and clinical tests of validity in measuring physical and mental health constructs. *Medical Care, 31*(3), 247–263.

95   Medical Outcomes Trust. (1990). *SF-36 (MOS 36 Item Short Form).* Boston, MA: Author.

96 Revicki, D. (1992). Relationship between health utility and psychometric health status measures. *Medical Care, 30*(5, S), MS274–282.

97 Rise, A., Kaplan, R., & Blumberg, E. (1991). Use of factor analysis to consolidate multiple outcome measures in COPD. *Journal of Clinical Epidemiology, 44*(6), 497–503.

98 Schrier, R., Burrow-Hudson, S. et al. (1994). Measuring, managing, and improving quality of life in end-stage renal disease. *American Journal of Kidney Disease, 24*(2), 383–388.

99 Tarlov, A., Ware, J., Greenfield, J. et al. (1989). The Medical Outcomes Study: An application of methods for monitoring results of medical care. *JAMA,* 262–925.

100 UDS~MR~^SM^ Policy for Release of Data. (1994). UDS~MR~^SM^ Subscriber News, *1*(2).

101 Velozo, C. (1994). Should occupational therapy choose a single functional outcome measure? *American Journal of Occupational Therapy, 48*(10), 946–947.

102 Ware, J.E., & Scherbourne, C.D. (1992). The MOS 36 item short-form health survey (SF-36): I. Conceptual framework and item selection. *Medical Care, 30*(6), 473–483.

103 Weiss, C. (1972). *Evaluation research: Methods for assessing program effectiveness.* Englewood Cliffs, NJ: Prentice-Hall.

104 Wellington, S., Benditsky, H., Tanitor, Z. et al. (1985). So you have a management information system: What's next? *Topics in Health Record Management, 5,* 53–63.

OUTCOME RESEARCH AND MEASUREMENT

105 Alexander, J.L., & Halstead, L.S. (1979). *Functional outcome assessment: A practical, new approach to follow-up.* 56th Annual Session of the American Congress of Rehabilitation Medicine, Honolulu, HI.

106 Anderson, T.P., McClure, W.J., Athelstan, G. et al. (1978). Stroke rehabilitation: Evaluation of its quality by assessing patient outcomes. *Archives of Physical Medicine and Rehabilitation, 59,* 170–185.

107 Balestra, D.J. (1992). Specialists or generalists? The Medical Outcomes Study. *JAMA, 268,* 1537–1538.

108 Bishop, D.S., Epstein, N.B., Keitner, G.I. et al. (1986). Stroke: Morale, family functioning, health status and functional capacity. *Archives of Physical Medicine and Rehabilitation, 67,* 84–87.

109 Black-Schaffer, R.M., Osberg, J.S. (1990). Return to work after stroke: Development of a predictive model. *Archives of Physical Medicine and Rehabilitation, 71,* 285–290.

110 Carey, R.G., Seibert, J.H., & Posavac, E.J. (1988). Who makes the most progress in inpatient rehabilitation? An analysis of functional gain. *Archives of Physical Medicine and Rehabilitation, 69,* 337–343.

111 Cummings, V., Kerner, J.F., Arones, S. et al. (1985). Day hospital service in rehabilitation medicine: An evaluation. *Archives of Physical Medicine and Rehabilitation, 66,* 86–91.

112 Davidoff, G.N., Keren, O., Ring, H. et al. (1991). Acute stroke patients: Long-term effects of rehabilitation and maintenance of gains. *Archives of Physical Medicine and Rehabilitation, 72,* 869–873.

113 Davies, A.R. (1994). *A guide to establishing programs and assessing outcomes in clinical settings.* Oakbrook Terrace, IL: Joint Commission on Accreditation of Healthcare Organizations.

114 DeFriese, G.H. (1990). Measuring the effectiveness of medical interventions: *New expectations of health services research. Health Services Research, 25*(5), 691–695.

115 Disler, P., Roy, R., & Smith, B. (1993). Predicting hours of care needed. *Archives of Physical Medicine and Rehabilitation, 74,* 139–143.

116 Feigenson, J.S., Githlow, H.S., & Greenberg, S.D. The disability oriented rehabilitation unit: A major factor influencing stroke outcome. *Stroke, 10,* 5–7.

117 Feinberg, S., Mackey, F., Steer, H., et al. (1979). Stroke outcome prediction by computer tomography. *Official Program of the American Academy of Physical Medicine and Rehabilitation,* 41st Annual Assembly, 77.

118 Fisher, A.G. (1992). Functional measures, part 1: What is function, what should we measure, and how should we measure it? *American Journal of Occupational Therapy, 46*(2), 183–185.

119 Forer, S.K., & Miller, L.S. (1980). Rehabilitation outcome: Comparative analysis of different patient types. *Archives of Physical Medicine and Rehabilitation, 61,* 359–365.

120 Forer, S.K., & Magnuson, R.I. Feedback reporting. (1984). In C. Granger & G. Gresham (Eds.), *Functional assessment in rehabilitation medicine* (pp. 171–193). Baltimore, MD: Williams and Wilkins.

121 Giacino, J.T., Kezmarsky, M.A., DeLuca, J., et al. (1991). Monitoring rate of recovery to predict outcome in minimally responsive patients. *Archives of Physical Medicine and Rehabilitation, 72,* 897–901.

122 Gilchrist, E., & Wilkinson, M. (1979). Some factors determining prognosis in young people with severe head injuries. *Archives of Neurology, 36,* 355–359.

123 Granger, C.V., Kaplan, M.T., Jones, B., et al. (1982). Stroke: Comparison of admissions in a community hospital. *Archives of Physical Medicine and Rehabilitation, 63,* 352–356.

124 Granger, C.V., & Gresham, G. (Eds.). *Functional assessment in medical rehabilitation.* Baltimore, MD: Williams and Wilkins.

125 Granger, C., Sotter, A., Hamilton, B., & Fiedler, R. (1993). Functional assessment scales: A study of persons after stroke. *Archives of Physical Medicine and Rehabilitation, 74,* 133–138.

126 Hertan, U.J., Dernopoulos, J., Yang, W., et al. (1984). Stroke rehabilitation: Correlation and prognostic value of computerized tomography and sequential functional assessment. *Archives of Physical Medicine and Rehabilitation, 65,* 505–508.

127 Hertan, J., & Yang, W. (1980). *Correlation and prognostic value of CT scan and Barthel Index in stroke rehabilitation.* Paper presented at the 42nd Annual Assembly of the American Academy of Physical Medicine and Rehabilitation, Washington, DC.

128 Holas, M., DePippo, K., & Reading, M. (1994). Aspiration and relative risk of medical complications following stroke. *Archives of Neurology, 51*(10), 1051–1053.

129   Jellinek, H.M., Torkelson, R., & Harvey, R. (1982). Functional abilities and distress levels in brain injured patients at long-term follow-up. *Archives of Physical Medicine and Rehabilitation, 63,* 160–162.

130   Johnston, M.V., & Keith, R.A. (1983). Cost–benefits of medical rehabilitation: Review and critique. *Archives of Physical Medicine and Rehabilitation, 64,* 147–154.

131   Johnston, M.V, & Keister, M. (1984). Early rehabilitation for stroke patients: A new look. *Archives of Physical Medicine and Rehabilitation, 65,* 437–441.

132   Johnston, M.V., & Miller, L.S. (1986). Cost-effectiveness of the Medicare three-hour regulation. *Archives of Physical Medicine and Rehabilitation, 67,* 581–584.

133   Johnston, M.V., Keith, R.A., & Hinderer, S.R. (1992). Measurement standards for interdisciplinary medical rehabilitation. [Special Education Issue]. *Archives of Physical Medicine and Rehabilitation, 73*(No 12-S).

134   Kaufer, J.M. (1983). Functional ability indices: Measurement problems in assessing their validity. *Archives of Physical Medicine and Rehabilitation, 64,* 260–267.

135   Keith, R.A. (1984). Functional assessment measures in medical rehabilitation: Current status. *Archives of Physical Medicine and Rehabilitation, 65,* 74–78.

136   Lehmann, J.F., Delateur, B.J., Fowler, R.S. et al. (1977). Stroke: Does rehabilitation affect outcome? *Archives of Physical Medicine and Rehabilitation, 56,* 375–382.

137   Malzer, R.L. (1988). Patient performance level during inpatient physical rehabilitation: Therapist, nurse, and patient perspectives. *Archives of Physical Medicine and Rehabilitation, 69,* 363–365.

138   McGinnis, G.E., Seward, M.L., DeJong, G. et al. (1986). Program evaluation of physical medicine and rehabilitation departments using self report Barthel. *Archives of Physical Medicine and Rehabilitation, 67,* 123–125.

139   Miller, L.S., & Forer, S.K. (1983). Mortality among stroke patients following rehabilitation. (Abstract). *Archives of Physical Medicine and Rehabilitation, 64,* 505.

140   Miller, L.S., & Johnston, M.V. (1985). One hundred point scale in functional assessment. (Abstract). *Archives of Physical Medicine and Rehabilitation, 66,* 556.

141   Miller, L.S., & Miyamoto, A.T. (1979). Computer tomography: Its potential as a predictor of functional recovery following stroke. *Archives of Physical Medicine and Rehabilitation, 60,* 108–109.

142   Miller, L.S., Miyamoto, A.T., & Forer, S.K. (1980). *The significance of carotid artery occlusion and stroke outcome.* Paper presented at the 42nd Annual Assembly of the American Academy of Physical Medicine and Rehabilitation, Washington, DC.

143   Mor, V., Granger, C.V., & Sherwood, C. (1983). Discharged rehabilitation patients: Impact of follow-up surveillance by friendly visitor. *Archives of Physical Medicine and Rehabilitation, 64,* 346–353.

144   Rappaport, M., Hall, K., Hopkins, K. et al. (1981). Evoked potential and head injury: Clinical applications. *Clinical Electroencephalography, 12,* 167–176.

145   Rao, N., Jellinek, H., Harvey, R. et al. (1984). Computerized tomography head scans as predictors of rehabilitation outcome. *Archives of Physical Medicine and Rehabilitation, 65,* 18–20.

146 Rao, N., Jellinek, H.M., & Woolston, D.C. (1985). Agitation in closed head injury: Haloperidol effects on rehabilitation outcome. *Archives of Physical Medicine and Rehabilitation, 66,* 30–34.

147 Reyes, R., & Heller, D. (1981). Traumatic head injury: Restlessness and agitation as prognosticators of physical and psychologic improvement in patients. *Archives of Physical Medicine and Rehabilitation, 62,* 20–23.

148 Robinson, R.G., Bolduc, P.L., & Kubos, K.L. (1985). Social functioning in stroke patients. *Archives of Physical Medicine and Rehabilitation, 66,* 496–500.

149 Rogers, J.C., & Holm, M.B. (1994). Accepting the challenge of outcomes research: Examining the effectiveness of occupational therapy practice. *American Journal of Occupational Therapy, 48*(10), 871–876.

150 Rondinelli, R.D., Murphy, J.R., Wilson, D.H. et al. (1991). Predictors of functional outcome and resource utilization in inpatient rehabilitation. *Archives of Physical Medicine and Rehabilitation, 72,* 447–452.

151 Schmidt, S.M., Herman, L.M., Koenig, P. et al. (1986). Status of stroke patients: A community assessment. *Archives of Physical Medicine and Rehabilitation, 67,* 99–102.

152 Scranton, J., Fogel, M., & Edman, W. (1975). Evaluation of functional levels of patients during and following rehabilitation. *Archives of Physical Medicine and Rehabilitation, 56,* 375–382.

153 Spettell, C.M., Ellis, D.W., Ross, S.E. et al. (1991). Time of rehabilitation admission and severity of trauma: Effect on brain injury outcome. *Archives of Physical Medicine and Rehabilitation, 72,* 320–325.

154 Timming, R., Orrison, W., & Mikula, J. (1982). Computerized tomography and rehabilitation outcomes after severe head trauma. *Archives of Physical Medicine and Rehabilitation, 63,* 154–159.

155 Udin, H., & May, B. (1982). *Rehabilitation: National norms and regional patterns of payment source and length of stay.* Paper presented as the 59th Annual Session of the American Congress of Rehabilitation Medicine, Houston, TX.

156 Weddell, R., Oddy, M., & Jenkins, D. (1980). Social adjustment after rehabilitation: A two year follow-up of patients with severe head injury. *Psychosocial Medicine, 10,* 257–263.

OUTPATIENT MEDICAL REHABILITATION OUTCOME MEASURES

157 Averill, R.F., Goldfield, H.I. et al. (1993, January). *Design and evaluation of a prospective payment system for ambulatory care.* Project sponsored by the Health Care Financing Administration, Office of Research and Demonstrations under cooperative agreement with the 3M Health Information Systems (Agreement No. 17-C-99369/1–02).

158 Benson, D.S. (1993). *Measuring outcomes in ambulatory care.* Chicago, IL: American Hospital Publishing.

159 Fairbanks, J., Davies, J. et al. (1980). The Owestry Low Back Pain Disability Questionnaire. *Physiotherapy, 66* (8), 271–274.

160 *Focus on Therapeutic Outcomes* (FOTO), Inc. (1993). Knoxville, TN.

161 Forer, S.K. (1994, July). *Guidelines for outcome measures and evaluation systems in outpatient rehabilitation.* Sacramento, CA: California Association of Rehabilitation Facilities, Outpatient Outcomes Task Force.

162 Forer, S.K. (1994, June). *Functional outcome measures in comprehensive outpatient rehabilitation programs.* Paper presented at the ACRM Symposium on Functional Outcome Measures. Minneapolis, MN.

163 Granger, C.V., & Wright B. (1993). Looking ahead to the use of functional assessment in ambulatory physiatric and primary care. *Physical Medicine and Rehabilitation Clinics of North America, 4*(3), 1–11.

164 Himmel, P.B. (1984). Functional assessment strategies in clinical medicine: The care of the arthritic patient. In *Functional assessment in rehabilitation medicine* (pp. 343–363). Baltimore, MD: Williams & Wilkins.

165 Lemsky, C., Miller, C. et al. (1991, November). *Reliability and validity of a physical performance and mobility examination for hospitalized elderly.* Paper presented at the annual meeting of the Gerontological Society of America, San Francisco, CA.

166 *Orthopedic Outcome System.* Chicago, IL: Formations in Health Care, Inc.

167 *RESTORE (Neuro Rehabilitation) Outcome System.* (1992). Chicago, IL: Formations in Health Care, Inc.

168 Tegner, Y., & Lysholm, J. (1985). Rating systems in the evaluation of knee ligament injuries. *Clinical Orthopedics and Related Research, 196,* 43–48.

169 Vernon, H., & Mior, S. (1991).The Neck Disability Index: A study of reliability and validity. *Journal of Manipulative and Physiological Therapeutics, 14* (7), 409–414.

PATIENT CLASSIFICATION AND PAYMENT SYSTEMS

170 Averill, R.F., Goldfield, H.I. et al. (1993, January). *Design and evaluation of a prospective payment system for ambulatory care.* Project sponsored by the Health Care Financing Administration, Office of Research and Demonstrations under cooperative agreement with the 3M Health Information Systems (agreement No. 17-C-99369/1–02).

171 Batavia, A.I., & DeJong, G. (1988). Prospective payment for medical rehabilitation: The DHHS report to Congress. *Archives of Physical Medicine and Rehabilitation, 69,* 377–380.

172 Costich, J.F. (1987). Acute care prospective payment: Impact on medical rehabilitation outcomes. Impact on medical rehabilitation outcomes. In M.J. Fuhrer (Ed.), *Rehabilitation outcomes: Analysis and measurement.* Baltimore, MD: Brookes Publishing.

173 DeJong, G. (1987). Medical rehabilitation outcome measurement in a changing health care market. In M.J. Fuhrer (Ed.), *Rehabilitation outcomes: Analysis and measurement.* Baltimore, MD: Brookes Publishing.

174 Harada, N., Kominiski, G., & Sofaer, S. (1993, Spring). Development of a resource-based patient classification scheme for rehabilitation. Blue Cross and Blue Shield Association: *Inquiry, 30,* 54–63.

175 Kane, R., Melvin, J., Hosek, S. et al. (1986). *Changes and outcomes for rehabilitative care: Implications for the prospective payment system* (Grant No. R-3424-HCFA). Report prepared for the Health Care Financing Administration, Santa Monica, CA : RAND Corp.

176 Muller, R., Nuzum, F.J., & Matthews, D. (1983). Inpatient medical rehabilitation: Results of the 1981 survey of hospitals and units. *Archives of Physical Medicine and Rehabilitation, 64,* 354–358.

177 National Association of Rehabilitation Facilities. (1985). *NARF position paper on a prospective payment system for inpatient medical rehabilitation services.* Washington, DC: Author.

178 American Rehabilitation Association. (1994, August). *Proposal for a Medicare prospective payment system for rehabilitation hospitals and units, expanding the conditions for exclusion from PPS, and rebasing of long term care hospitals.* Washington, DC: Author.

179 Osberg, J.S., Haley, S.M., McGinnis, G.E. et al. (1990). Characteristics of cost outliers who did not benefit from stroke rehabilitation. *American Journal of Physical Medicine and Rehabilitation, 69*(3), 117–125.

180 Department of Health and Human Services, Health Care Financing Administration. (1994, December). Request for Proposal (RFP) No. HCFA-95-012/PK for *Evaluation of case classification systems and a design of a prospective payment model for inpatient rehabilitation.* Baltimore, MD: Author.

181 Stineman, M., Dejong, G., Escare, J. et al. (1992). *Developing a classification for medical rehabilitation: Predicting LOS/charges and outcomes.* Washington, DC: National Association of Rehabilitation Facilities.

182 Stinemen, M.G., Escare, J. et al. (1994, April). A case-mix classification system for medical rehabilitation. *Medical Care, 23*(4), 366–378.

183 Stineman, M.G., Hamilton, B. et al. (1994). Four methods of characterizing disability in the formation of function related groups. *Archives of Physical Medicine and Rehabilitation, 74,* 1277–1283.

184 Tepper, S., DeJong, G. et al. (1995). Criteria for selection of a payment method for inpatient medical rehabilitation. *Archives of Physical Medicine and Rehabilitation, 76,* 349–354.

185 Wilkerson, D., Batavia, A., & DeJong, G. (1992). Use of functional status measures for payment of medical rehabilitation services. *Archives of Physical Medicine and Rehabilitation, 73,* 111–120.

PROGRAM EVALUATION

186 Breckenridge, K. (1978). Medical rehabilitation program evaluation. *Archives of Physical Medicine and Rehabilitation, 59,* 419–423.

187 Commission on Accreditation of Rehabilitation Facilities. (1979, December). *Program evaluation in inpatient medical rehabilitation facilities.* Tuscon, AZ: Author.

188 Forer, S.K. (1981, November). Integrating program evaluation and quality assurance. *Journal of the Organization of Rehabilitation Evaluators, 2,* 15–21.

189 Forer, S.K., & Everette, J. (1989). Utilization of program evaluation and quality assurance for marketing: The California experience. In B. England, R.M. Glass, & C.H. Patterson (Eds.), *Quality rehabilitation: Results oriented patient care* (pp. 95–101). Chicago, IL: American Hospital Publishing.

190 Forer, S.K. (1992). How to make program evaluation work for you: Utilization for program service management. *NeuroRehabilitation: An Interdisciplinary Journal, 2*(4), 52–71.

191 Franklin, J.L., & Thrasher, J.H. (1976). *An introduction to program evaluation.* New York: Wiley.

192 Lorber, C., & Lundstrom, J.S. (1981, August). Managing staff resistance to program evaluation. *Journal of the Organization of Rehabilitation Evaluators, 1,* 19–33.

193 Wilkerson, D.L. (1991). Program and outcome evaluation: Opportunity for the 1990's. *Occupational Therapy Practice, 2*(2), 1–15.

PSYCHIATRIC REHABILITATION OUTCOME MEASURES

194 American Association for Partial Hospitalization. (1994). *AAPH Outcomes Project. Client Satisfaction Questionnaire.* Alexandria, VA: Author.

195 American Psychiatric Association. (1987). Global Assessment of Functioning. In *Diagnostic and statistical manual of mental disorders* (3rd ed.). Washington, DC: Author.

196 Farkas, M., & Anthony, W.A. Outcome analysis in psychiatric rehabilitation. In M.J. Fuhrer (Ed.), *Rehabilitation outcomes: Analysis and measurement.* Baltimore, MD: Brookes Publishing.

197 Feragne, M., Longabauch, R., & Stevenson, J. (1983). The psychosocial functioning inventory. *Evaluation and the Health Professionals, 6,* 25–48.

198 Folstein, J.M., Folstein, S.E., & McHugh, P.R. (1975). Mini-mental state. A practical method for grading the cognitive state of patients for the clinician. *Journal of Psychiatric Research, 12,* 189–198.

199 Guy, M., & Moore, L. (1982, June). The goal attainment scale for psychiatric inpatients. *Quality Review Bulletin,* pp. 19–29.

200 King, R., Houghland, J., Shephard, J., & Gallagher, E. (1980). Organizational effects on mentally retarded adults: A longitudinal analysis. *Evaluation of the Health Professionals, 3,* 85–101.

201 Lawton, M.P., & Brody E.M. (1969). Assessment of older people. Self-maintaining and instrumental activities of daily living. *Gerontology, 9,* 179–186.

202 McLean Hospital Evaluation Service Unit. *BASIS-32.* Belmont, MA: Author.

203 Medical Outcomes Trust. (1990). *SF (MOS 36 Item Short Form).* Boston, MA: Author.

204 American Association for Partial Hospitalization. (1994). *Outcomes Measurement Protocol.* Alexandria, VA: Author.

205 University Associates in Psychiatry. (1991). *Child Behavior Checklist.* Burlington, VT: Author.

206 University of Minnesota, Family Social Science Department. (1985). *FACES III.* St. Paul, MN: Author.

207 Yesavage, J. et al. (1983). Development and validation of a geriatric depression screening scale. *Journal of Psychiatric Research, 17,* 37–49.

QUALITY MANAGEMENT & QUALITY IMPROVEMENT

208 American Congress of Rehabilitation Medicine—Head Injury ISIG. (1993). *Survey of important outcome objectives and measurement systems for TBI: Payor and provider perspectives.* Skokie, IL: Author.

209 Bartilotta, K., & Rzasa, C.B. (1982). Quality assurance utilizing a computerized patient information system. *Quality Review Bulletin, 8*(3), 17–22.

210 Condeluci, A., Ferris, L., & Bogdan, A. (1992). Outcome and value. The survivor perspective. *Journal of Head Trauma Rehabilitation, 7*(4), 37–45.

211 Evaluating quality of patient care: A strategy relating outcome. (1971). *Journal of the American Medical Association, 218*(4): 564–569.

212 Evans, R., & Ruff, R. (1992). Outcome and value: A perspective on rehabilitation outcomes achieved in acquired brain injury. *Journal of Head Trauma Rehabilitation, 7*(4), 24–36.

213 Johnston, M., Wilkerson, D., & Maney, M. (1993). Evaluation of the quality and outcomes of medical rehabilitation programs. In J.A. Delisa (Ed.), *Rehabilitation medicine: Principles and practice* (pp. 240–268). Philadelphia, PA: Lippincott.

214 Joint Commission on Accreditation of Healthcare Organizations. (1994). *Improving organizational performance.* Oakbrook, IL: Author.

215 Papasptra, R. (1992). Outcome and value following brain injury: A financial payers perspective. *Journal of Head Trauma Rehabilitation, 7*(4), 11–23.

216 Pollak, V., Pesce, A., & Kant, K. (1992, June 19) Continuous quality improvement in chronic disease: A computerized medical record enables descriptions of a severity index to evaluate outcomes in end-stage renal disease. *American Journal of Kidney Diseases,* 514–522.

217 National Association of Rehabilitation Facilities. (1994). *Final Report of the RQI Network Evaluation Study.* Reston, VA: Rehabilitation Research and Education Fund (RREF), and the American Rehabilitation Association.

SPINAL CORD INJURY OUTCOME MEASURES

218 American Spinal Injury Association. (1982). *Standard for neurological classification of SCI patients.* Chicago, IL: Author.

219 Alexander, J., & Fuhrer, M.J. (1984). Functional assessment of individuals with physical impairments. In A.S. Halper & M.J. Fuhrer (Eds.), *Functional assessment in rehabilitation* (pp. 45–59). Baltimore, MD: Brookes Publishing.

220 Fuhrer, M., Rintala, D., Hart, K., Clearman, R., & Young, M. (1992). Relationship of life satisfaction to impairment, disability, and handicap among persons with spinal cord injury living in the community. *Archives of Physical Medicine and Rehabilitation, 73,* 424–430.

221 Rintala, D.H. et al. (1984). Self-observation and reporting technique (SORT): Description and clinical application. In M.J. Fuhrer (Ed.), *Functional assessment in rehabilitation* (pp. 205–221). Baltimore, MD: Brookes Publishing.

222   Sevick, M., Zucconi, S. et al. (1992, November 1). Characteristics and health service utilization patterns of ventilator-dependent patients cared for within a vertically integrated health system. *American Journal of Critical Care,* 45–51.

223   Whiteneck, G. et al. (1992). Quantifying handicap: A new measure of long-term rehabilitation outcomes. *Archives of Physical Medicine and Rehabilitation, 73,* 519–526.

224   Whiteneck, G. (1987). Outcome analysis in spinal cord injury rehabilitation. In M.J. Fuhrer (Ed.), *Rehabilitation outcomes: Analysis and measurement.* Baltimore, MD: Brookes Publishing.

SUBACUTE OUTCOME MEASURES (REHABILITATION AND MEDICAL)

225   Albert, M., & Cohen, C. (1992). The Test for Severe Impairment: An instrument for the assessment of patients with severe cognitive dysfunction. *Journal of the American Geriatrics Society, 40*(5), 449–453.

226   Dracup, K., Walden, J., Stevenson, L., & Brecht, M. (1992). Quality of life in patients with advanced heart failure. *Journal of Heart and Lung Transplantation,* 11(2,1), 273–279.

227   Duguette, R., Dupius, G., & Perrault, J. (1994). A new approach for quality of life assessment in cardiac patients: Rationale and validation of the Quality of Life Systemic Inventory. *Canadian Journal of Cardiology, 10*(1), 106–112.

228   Forer, S.K., & Wall, T. (1994, September). Quality and outcome management: Strategies for subacute providers. Guest column in *Subacute Care Management.* Atlanta, GA: American Health Consultants.

229   Forer, S.K., & Shumacker, P. (1994, November). Quality and outcomes management: Strategies for subacute providers. *JCAHO Long Term Care Update.*

230   Forer, S.K. (1995, June/July). Outcome and quality management in subacute care. *Rehabilitation management.* Marina Del Ray, CA: CurAnt Communications.

231   Formations in Health Care, Inc. (1994, Winter). New measurement tool will enhance subacute competitiveness. *Physical Rehabilitation Update, 3*(2), 1–4. [Newsletter published by Formations in Health Care, Chicago, IL.]

232   Kramer, A., et al. (1993). *A policy study of the cost-effectiveness of institutional sub-acute care alternatives and services.* Project funded by the Health Care Financing Administration (HCFA), Department of Health and Human Services (Contract No. 18-C-99491/8/01). Denver, CO: Center for Health Services Research, University of Colorado Health Sciences Center.

233   Lareau, S.C., Carrieri-Kohlman, V., Janson-Bjerklie, S., & Roos, P. (1994). Development and testing of the Pulmonary Functional Status and Dyspnea Questionnaire (PFSDQ). *Heart and Lung, 23*(3), 242–250.

234   Leiter, P., & Sipes, C. (1995). *Medical Outcome System: Subacute Medical Outcome Instrument.* Chicago, IL: Formations in Health Care, Inc.

235   Linn, N.M., Gurel L., & Linn, B.S. (1977). Patient outcome as a measure of quality of nursing home care. *American Journal of Public Health, 67,* 337–344.

236   Minimum Data Set (MDS) for Nursing Home Resident Assessment and Care Screening. (1992, December 28). *Federal Register, 57*(249), 61615–61733.

237   Naessen, J., Leibson, C., Krishan, I., & Ballard, D. (1992, December). Contribution of a measure of disease complexity (COMPLEX) to prediction of outcome and charges among hospitalized patients. *Mayo Clinic Proceedings, 67*(12), 1140–1149.

238   Osterweil, D., Mulford, P., Syndulko, K., & Martin, M. (1994). Cognitive function in old and very old patients in a residential facility: Relationship of age, education and dementia. *Journal of American Geriatrics Society, 42*(7), 766–773.

239   Siu, A., Reuben, D., Ouslander, J., & Osterweil, D. (1993). Using multidimensional health measures in older persons to identify risk of hospitalization and skilled nursing placement. *Quality of Life Research, 2*(4), 253–261.

240   Tedesco, C., Manning, S., Lindsay, R., Alexander, C., Owen, R., & Smucker, M. (1990). Functional assessment of elderly patients after percutaneous aortic balloon valvuloplasty: New York Heart Association Classification vs. functional status questionnaire. *Heart and Lung, 19*(2), 118–125.

241   Tresch, D., Neahring, J., Duthie, E. et al. (1993). Outcomes of cardiopulmonary resuscitation in nursing homes: Can we predict who will benefit. *American Journal of Medicine, 95*(2), 123–130.

242   Uniform Data System for Medical Rehabilitation. (1994, October). UDS$_{MR}$^{SM} subacute services expand. *UDS$_{MR}$ Update, 8*(4).

243   Vibbert, S. (1992). *Medical outcomes and guidelines sourcebook.* Washington, DC: Faulkner & Gray.

UNIFORM TERMINOLOGY AND CONCEPTUAL FRAMEWORK

244   American Occupational Therapy Association. (1995). *Uniform Terminology for Occupational Therapy* (3rd ed.). Bethesda, MD: Author.

245   World Health Organization. (1980). *International Classification of Impairments, Disabilities and Handicaps.* Geneva, Switzerland: Author.

VOCATIONAL REHABILITATION OUTCOME MEASURES

246   Bolton, B. (1987). Outcome analysis in vocational rehabilitation. In M.J. Fuhrer (Ed.), *Rehabilitation outcomes: Analysis and measurement.* Baltimore, MD: Brookes Publishing.

247   Crewe, N.M., & Athelstan, G.T. (1981). Functional assessment in vocational rehabilitation: A system approach to diagnosis and goal setting. *Archives of Physical Medicine and Rehabilitation, 62,* 299–305.

248   Gibson, D., Weis, D., Dawes, R., & Lofquist, H. (1970). *Manual for the Minnesota Satisfaction Scales.* (Minnesota Studies in Vocation Rehabilitation, 27). Minneapolis, MN: Vocational Psych Research, University of Minnesota.

249   Kravetz, S., Florian, V., & Wright, G. (1985). The development of a multifaceted measure of rehabilitation effectiveness. Theoretical rational and scale construction. *Rehabilitation Psychology, 30,* 195–208.

250   Rossler, R., & Bolton, B. (1983). Assessment and enhancement of functional vocational capabilities: A five year research strategy. *Vocational Evaluation and Work Adjustment Bulletin* (Monograph 11).

251 Institute for Personality and Ability Testing. (1985). *Manual for Form E (16 PF-E) The Sixteen Personality Factor Questionnaire.*

252 Tinsley, H., Warnken, R., Weis, D., Dawes, R., & Lofquist, L. (1970). *A follow-up survey of former clients in the Minnesota Division of VR.* (Minnesota Studies in Vocation Rehabilitation, 26). Minneapolis, MN: Vocational Psych Research, University of Minnesota.

253 Weis, W. (1981). Independent behavior and moral judgment in primary public schools. *Psychologic in Erziehund Unterrich, 28*(6), 334–343.

254 Westerheide, W., & Lenhart, L. (1973). Development and reliability of a pretest-posttest rehabilitation services outcome measure. *Rehabilitation Research and Practice Review, 4*(3), 15–24.

APPENDICES

APPENDIX A.
PROGRAM EVALUATION SYSTEM
FOR COMPREHENSIVE INPATIENT REHAB

PRIMARY OBJECTIVE	RECOMMENDED MEASURE(S)	WHO APPLIED TO	TIME OF MEASURE	DATA SOURCE	EXPECTANCY Min.	Goal	Opt.
1. Maximize Functional Independence	Average FIM gain from admission to discharge	All General Rehab patients who complete program	Adm. to disch.	Patient ratings	**19**	**23**	**27**
	a) Stroke				20	24	28
	b) Neuro				17	20	23
	c) Arthritis/Amputee/Ortho				16	20	25
	d) Other				15	20	25
2. Avoid Institutionalization	Percent of patients returning to non-institutional settings (home,	All General Rehab patients (excluding short term evals.)	Discharge & 6 months post D/C.	Medical Record, follow-up interview.	70	80	90
3. Maximize Service Efficiency	LOS Efficiency (average FIM Gain/LOS)	All General Rehab patients (excluding short term evals.)	Admission to Discharge	Patient ratings, LOS	.90	1.25	1.6
4. Optimize Program LOS	Average LOS < UDS Nat.	All General Rehab patients who complete program	Admission & Discharge	Medical Records Records	**24**	**21**	**18**
	a) Stroke				24	21	18
	b) Neuro				24	20	16
	c) Arthritis/Amputee/Ortho				22	18	14
	d) Other				23	20	17
5. Increase Self-Care Skills	Average gain in Self Care admit to discharge (6 items)	All General Rehab patients who complete program	Adm., D/C & 6 months post D/C	Patient ratings, follow-up evals., telephone.	**1.2**	**1.4**	**1.6**
	a) Stroke				1.2	1.5	1.8
	b) Neuro				1.0	1.3	1.6
	c) Arthritis/Amputee/Ortho				1.0	1.3	1.6
	d) Other				1.2	1.5	1.8
6. Increase Mobility Skills	Average gain in Mobility admit to discharge (5 items)	All General Rehab patients who complete program	Adm., D/C & 6 months post D/C	Patient ratings, follow-up evals., telephone.	**1.5**	**1.8**	**2.1**
	a) Stroke				1.5	1.8	2.1
	b) Neuro				1.5	1.8	2.2
	c) Arthritis/Amputee/Ortho				1.4	1.8	2.2
	d) Other				1.4	1.7	2.0

	Indicator	Population	Timing	Method			
7. Maximize Bowel & Bladder Management	Percent at level 4 or above by discharge.	All General Rehab patients who complete program	Adm., D/C, & 6 months post d/c.	Patient ratings, follow-up evals., telephone	70	80	90
8. Increase Communication Skills	Average gain in communication from admission to discharge	All stroke patients receiving speech therapy	Adm., D/C, & 6 months post d/c	Patient ratings, follow-up evals., and telephone	0.5	0.7	0.9
9. Maximize Patient/Family Satisfaction	Percent satisfied with overall program	All General Rehab patients who complete program	2 weeks post d/c	Mailed survey or telephone interview	70	80	90
10. Maintain Functional Gains	Percent of patients who maintain or improve FIM scores from discharge to follow-up.	All General Rehab patients who complete program	D/C, 2 and 6 months post D/C.	Patient ratings, follow-up evals., telephone	70	80	90
11. Minimize Program Interruptions Due to Medical Complications	Percent of patients transferred back to acute for medical reasons.	All General Rehab patients admitted to Rehab.	Adm. to Disch.	Medical Record	10	5	0

APPENDIX B.
PROGRAM EVALUATION MODEL SUBACUTE REHAB.

PRIMARY OBJECTIVE	RECOMMENDED) MEASURE(S)	WHO APPLIED TO	TIME OF MEASURE	DATA SOURCE SOURCE	EXPECTANCY Min.	Goal	Opt.
1. Maximize Functional Independence	Average FIM gain admit to discharge a) Stroke b) Orthopedic c) Other Rehab	All Subacute patients (excluding short stay < 7 days)	Adm., D/C & 6 months post d/c	Patient ratings, follow-up evals., and telephone	**17** 18 15 14	**22** 22 22 17	**26** 26 29 20
2. Avoid Institutionalization	Percent of patients returning to non-institutional settings.	All Subacute patients (excluding patients transferred to acute rehab)	Adm. to disch.	Medical Record	65	75	85
3. Minimize Medical Complications	Percent of patients transferred back to acute for medical reasons.	All Subacute patients	Adm. to D/C	Medical Record	20	12	4
4. Maximize Service Efficiency	LOS Efficiency (Average FIM gain/LOS)	All Subacute patients	Adm. - disch.	Patient ratings, medical record	0.5	0.8	1.1
5. Optimize Program LOS	Average LOS < Nat. avg a) Stroke b) Orthopedic c) Other Rehab	All Subacute patients (excluding short term evals.)	Adm. - disch.	Medical record	**22** 26 20 24	**18** 23 16 19	**14** 20 12 14
6. Contain Program Costs	Average cost per day	All Subacute patients	Adm. - disch.	Patient Accounts	525	450	375
7. Maximize Patient/Family Satisfaction	Percent satisfied with overall program	All Subacute patients who complete program	2 weeks post d/c	Mailed survey or telephone	70	80	90
8. Maximize Bowel and Bladder Management	Percent at level 3 or above by discharge	All Subacute Stroke patients	Discharge	Patient ratings, medical record	65	75	85

9. Increase Self-Care Skills	Average gain in Self-Care admit to discharge a) Stroke b) Orthopedic c) Other Rehab	All Subacute patients	Adm., D/C & 6 months post d/c	Patient ratings, follow-up evals., telephone	**1.0** 1.0 1.0 0.9	**1.2** 1.2 1.3 1.2	**1.4** 1.4 1.6 1.5
10. Increase Mobility Skills	Average gain in Mobility admit to discharge a) Stroke b) Orthopedic c) Other Rehab	All Subacute patients	Adm., D/C, & 6 months post d/c	Patient ratings, follow-up evals., telephone interviews	**1.2** 1.2 1.3 1.1	**1.5** 1.5 1.6 1.4	**1.8** 1.8 1.9 1.7
11. Maintain Functional Gains	Percent of patients who maintain or improve FIM scores after discharge	All Sub-acute patients (excluding short term evals < 7 days)	6 months post d/c	Patient Self-report report, telephone interviews	65	75	85
12. Appropriate Level of Care Utilization	Percent of Sub-acute patients who require: < 1 hr. of therapy & < 4 hrs. nursing care OR > 2.5 hrs. therapy & > 5.5 hrs. nursing care	All Sub-acute patients	Adm. - disch.	Level of care determination (UR audits)	75	85	95

APPENDIX C.
PROGRAM EVALUATION SYSTEM FOR OUTPATIENT REHAB.

PRIMARY OBJECTIVE	RECOMMENDED MEASURE(S)	WHO APPLIED TO	TIME OF MEASURE	DATA SOURCE	EXPECTANCY Min.	Goal	Opt.
1. Maximize Patient/Family Satisfaction	Percent satisfied with O/P program	All patients responding to questionnaire	2 weeks post d/c	Mailed survey or telephone interview	75	85	95
2. Maximize Mobility Skills	FAM, RESTORE or APG's/PECS	All outpatients who complete program	D/C & 6 months post d/c	Patient ratings, follow-up evals., and telephone interviews	1.2	1.5	1.8
3. Maximize Self–Care Skills	FAM, RESTORE or APG's/PECS	All outpatients who complete program	D/C & 6 months post d/c	Patient ratings, follow-up evals., and telephone interviews	1.1	1.4	1.7
4. Maximize Communication	FAM, RESTORE or APG's/PECS	All outpatients who received Speech	D/C & 6 months post d/c	Patient ratings, follow-up evals., and telephone interviews	0.9	1.2	1.5
5. Assure appropriate provision of care	Percent of patients whose Tx goals were appropriate to diagnosis	All outpatients who complete program	Adm	Peer review of treatment plans	80	90	100
6. Minimize Number of Inappropriate Referrals	Percent of inappropriate referrals	All outpatients	Determined by 2nd visit	Clinical assessment	20	10	0
7. Assure timeliness of Tx.	Percent of O/P's whose Tx was initiated within 72 hrs. of authorization	All outpatients with Tx. authorization	1st. Tx visit	Documentation review	80	90	100
8. Maximize Return to Work	Percent of patients who return to work and/or enter vocational rehab.	All patients who were working prior to injury or were in school	3 & 6 months post D/C	Mailed survey or or telephone interview	75	85	95

9. Assure appropriate case management	Plan for follow–up care and communication with referring MD	All outpatients who complete program	2 weeks post discharge	Documentation review and MD interview	75	85	95
10. Minimize Preventable Medical Complications	Percent of patients who develop medical complications related to injury requiring intervention	All outpatients who complete program	3 & 6 months post D/C	Patient/family self report	20	10	0

INDEX